Support

You become the rock of support
upon which your loved one clings.

Clinging to the support you provide,
she can flourish even in the midst
of her journey through breast cancer.

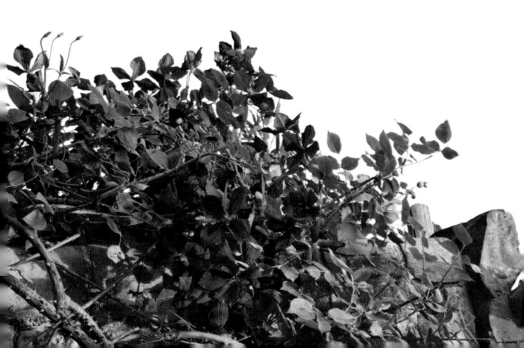

Breast Cancer Support Partner Handbook

Tips for Becoming an Effective Support Partner

Judy C. Kneece, RN, OCN

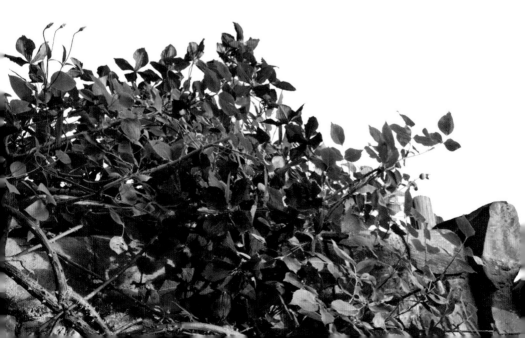

Understanding the Vital Role of Your Support

"Vines need cool roots, lots of sun for optimal growing conditions and, obviously, something to grow on—they need a trellis or arbor to flourish."

—*The Consulting Gardener*

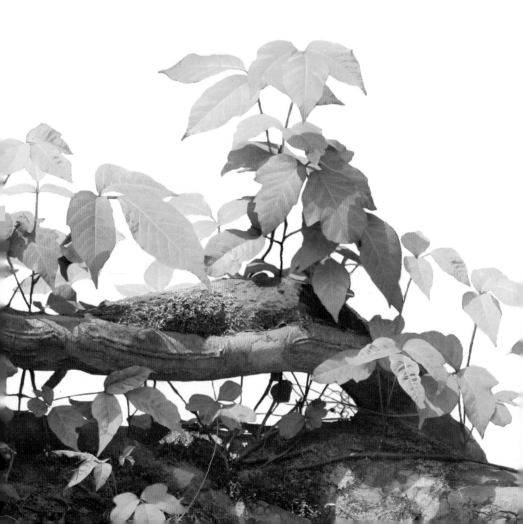

*A*fter a cancer diagnosis, patients and support partners share survival characteristics similar to a vine and trellis. Both endure and grow when the right elements are provided. However, without these necessary elements, they fail to thrive.

Cool Roots

A vine's roots require that the temperature of the soil stay cool. A patient requires the environmental climate she inhabits (lives in) to stay emotionally cool. If it does not, it will be very difficult to thrive emotionally.

Lots of Sun

Vines are dependent on the warm light of the sun on a regular schedule to allow them to receive the nutrients needed for growth. Patients need the outside warmth of support and caring from someone on a regular basis to find the strength to endure the challenges a cancer diagnosis brings.

Something to Grow On

Vines need a trellis, arbor, tree, rock or other stable object on which to grow. Vines cling to this object of support for additional growth to occur. The stable object provides the environment most conducive for growth. Without an object on which to grow, the vine branches would be forced to remain on the ground to endure the moisture and extreme changes that occur. This environment would cause the vine to fail to bloom and prevent it from bringing forth its potential beauty. Only when a vine has a stable object to cling to which provides support for its growth will its beauty be fully manifested.

Patients also thrive when there is someone they can cling to. Someone who provides them a place to rest emotionally and shelters them from the harsh environment a cancer diagnosis can bring. With someone beside them, acting as a supporting trellis, they are allowed to continue their growth, even during hard times, reaching their full potential and flourishing.

Because of their supporting environment, support partners become the trellis, rock or arbor that allows patients to flourish, in spite of the adverse challenges cancer presents.

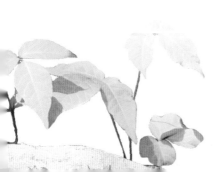

7th Edition 2010; Revised 6th Edition 2007; Fully Revised 5th Edition 2003; 4th Revised Edition 2001; 3rd Revised Edition 1999; 2nd Edition 1997; 1st Edition 1995.
ISBN 978-1-886665-24-8
Library of Congress Card Number: 2009941888
Printed in the United States of America
Published by EduCare Publishing Inc.

To order:

EduCare
3294 Ashley Phosphate Road, Suite 1-A
North Charleston, SC 29418
1-800-849-9271 or Fax: 843-760-6988
www.educareinc.com or www.breasthealthcare.com

Illustrations: Debra Strange, Setsuko Lawson

Publisher's Cataloging-In-Publication Data
(Prepared by The Donohue Group, Inc.)

Kneece, Judy C.
   [Helping your mate face breast cancer.]
   Breast cancer support partner handbook : tips for becoming an effective support partner /Judy C. Kneece. -- 7th ed.
      p. : ill. ; cm.
   Originally published as: Helping your mate face breast cancer : tips for becoming an effective support partner for the one you love during the breast cancer experience.
   Includes bibliographical references and index.
   ISBN: 978-1-886665-24-8

1. Breast--Cancer--Patients. 2. Cancer--Patients--Family relationships. I. Title.
RC280.B8 K569 2010
362.1/9699449   2009941888

Dedication

This book is dedicated to all of the patients and their support partners who have shared openly and honestly about their physical and emotional journeys with breast cancer. Their courage serves as a source of inspiration and proof that facing a crisis together can make a relationship even more meaningful and fulfilling.

A special debt of gratitude is extended to Cindy Dreher, MPH, MAT, for her visionary efforts in women's health issues by recognizing the acute need for the psychosocial support of patients and their families during the breast cancer experience. It is through her personal support that I had the opportunity to develop a psychosocial program to meet this need. Her influence is evident throughout this book and in my work with breast cancer patients.

To Tom Winnett, I owe my motivation to begin programs for the support partner. After speaking to a large group of women, Tom looked at me with tears in his eyes and said, *"Women have many places to go for help, but where is a man supposed to get help? … We hurt, too."* Thanks, Tom, for being frank and acting as a catalyst for including the support partner and family in all of my work as a Breast Health Navigator. From Tom's expressed need, I started a group for support partners of breast cancer patients.

To my husband, Dr. Robert Karl Hetz, who became my support partner after I recently fell and broke all of the bones in my ankle and required care for three months. From this experience of suddenly becoming unable to care for myself, I can now say with firm conviction that his role as a support partner was as important as any medical care I received. His presence, physical care, advocacy for my needs to the healthcare team and words of encouragement significantly eased the burden of the long days of bed rest, immobility and many weeks of physical therapy as I learned to walk again.

My final dedication is to all of the support partners who have shared openly with me about their fears, emotional pain, challenges and triumphs experienced in their new role. This book reflects their journey as retold to me as their Breast Cancer Navigator. Without a doubt, I can say that an effective supportive partner is as needed as any medical treatment we can provide for a newly diagnosed breast cancer patient.

Acknowledgements

A special word of appreciation to the following people for their contributions to this work:

Calvin Chao, MD, Director, Medical Affairs, Genomic Health, Inc.

Anna Cluxton, MBA, Survivor; President, Young Survival Coalition, Columbus, Ohio

Edward P. Dalton, MD, FACS, Elliot Hospital Breast Center, Manchester, New Hampshire; Past President, National Consortium of Breast Centers

Jennifer L. Harper, MD, Assistant Professor of Radiation Oncology, Medical University of South Carolina

Robert Karl Hetz, MD, Family Practice, Charleston, South Carolina

Kevin Hughes, MD, FACS, Surgical Director, Avon Foundation Comprehensive Breast Evaluation Center, Massachusetts General; Co-Director, Breast and Ovarian Cancer Genetics and Risk Assessment Program; Assistant Professor of Surgery, Harvard Medical School

George P. Keogh, MD, Medical Oncologist, Charleston Hematology Oncology Associates, Charleston, South Carolina

Rosemary Lambert-Falls, MD, Medical Oncologist, Columbia, South Carolina

Lisa Martinez, RN, BSNM, JD, Survivor, Founder and Executive Director of The Women's Sexual Health Foundation, Cleveland, Ohio

Maurice Nahabedian, MD, FACS, Associate Professor of Plastic Surgery, Georgetown University, Washington, DC

John S. Ravita, MD, FACRO, Medical Director, Georgia Center for Total Cancer Care at Cowles Clinic, Greensboro, Georgia

Ervin Shaw, MD, Chief of Pathology, Lexington Medical Center, West Columbia, South Carolina

Al Barrineau, Krystle Brown-Shaw, and *Brian Cluxton,* Support Partners, for their commentaries on their experiences during their loved one's breast cancer

Debra Strange and *Setsuko Lawson,* Medical Illustrators

Bianca Schumacher, Graphic Design and Layout

Mindy Wilson, Project Manager, Editorial Services

Jerri White and *Saralyn White,* Editorial Services

Table of Contents

About the Author

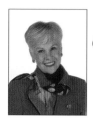

Judy C. Kneece, RN, OCN, is a certified oncology nurse with a specialty in breast cancer. She began her career as a Breast Health Navigator in a hospital where she developed her concept of patient navigation. In 1994, she started EduCare Inc. to train other nurses as Breast Health Navigators and to write educational information for breast cancer patients.

During the past fifteen years, EduCare Inc. has been a leader in developing educational materials and in training nurses to support breast cancer patients. Judy has trained over 2,000 registered nurses to fill the Breast Health Navigator role in hospitals, breast centers and physicians' offices. Over 500 hospitals and breast centers have used her Comprehensive Strategic Planning principles to implement breast care programs that emphasize pre-treatment interdisciplinary care conferences and the role of the Nurse Navigator.

The first edition of this book was published in 1995 and served as a pioneer in the area of addressing the unique needs of breast cancer support partners. Over 220,000 patients have used the companion book, *Breast Cancer Treatment Handbook,* as their recovery guide through breast cancer. Judy has authored three other books about breast care and created a set of 367 *Breast Health Teaching Sheets* designed to help nurses and doctors support and educate their patients.

Her background working in a hospital as a Breast Health Navigator gave her new insights into the needs of women and their families going through breast cancer. She has also intensely researched the breast cancer experience and the needs of patients and families through focus groups.

Judy presently serves as a national consultant for breast centers and hospitals. She serves as a member of the American College of Surgeons' Education Committee for the National Accreditation Program for Breast Centers (NAPBC) and on the advisory board for the Clinical Breast Care Project. She has served as a contributing editor for numerous national women's magazines on the issues of breast health and cancer and has over 40 nationally published articles on breast care topics. Judy speaks widely to patients on triumphant survivorship.

The Voices of Experience

When I finished writing this manuscript, it was not really complete. It lacked the voice of experience—a peer who had actually lived through the experience. You, a new support partner, needed to hear from someone who had personally experienced the same feelings, fears, challenges and joys of the inherited support partner role. My experience has been in the role as a coach for patients and their support partners, offering professional support by helping them to identify the challenges ahead and to develop skills to best deal with them. To offer you the experience of a peer, I have asked three support partners to share their perspectives on a variety of topics.

Sprinkled throughout this book are their feelings about the intimate experiences they faced during their support partner role. It is our hope that the sharing of their personal journeys will give you the courage to know that you and the one you love are not alone. Others have faced the same challenges and managed to face this unexpected life crisis, using it as a time to grow closer emotionally. It is not an easy process, but it is achievable. I want to introduce you to three support partners, Al Barrineau, Krystle Brown-Shaw and Brian Cluxton.

Al Barrineau — Support Partner

I had the privilege of working with Al and his wife, Harriett, for three years in the early 1990s, as they worked through the breast cancer experience. Involved with them in their journey were four sons, who were then ages 14 to 21.

Harriett was diagnosed with a large tumor that required a mastectomy. Eventually, she underwent a second mastectomy and bilateral reconstruction. During this time they were active in support groups, sharing their pain during their journey while offering encouragement to others. Harriett has served as a Reach to Recovery volunteer, and they both remained active in support groups for several years.

Al has shared his challenges and struggles with many other spouses. Throughout this book he reveals many of his feelings and experiences with you. Harriett provides the same commentary for the patient's book, the *Breast Cancer Treatment Handbook*.

Krystle Brown-Shaw — Support Partner

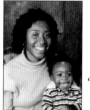

Krystle was a young woman who had just completed years of schooling, embarked on a new career and had become a new mom when her own mom, Earnestine Brown, was diagnosed with breast cancer.

"I was there when Mom came out of the doctor's office and told me she had breast cancer. 'Shocked' was my first response! This was my mom—the person who had always taken care of my siblings and me. Now it was my turn. She needed me. What could I do to help her?" Like all support partners, Krystle inherited her role because of her close relationship to the newly diagnosed patient.

As one of three siblings who had been raised in a single parent home, there was never any doubt in Krystle's mind as to her response to her mom's diagnosis. Her mom had worked two jobs to send Krystle and her siblings to school and had always been the strong one in the family. Now role reversal was in order. Her mom was the one who needed support.

Her mom underwent a lumpectomy with lymph node dissection, chemotherapy and radiation therapy. Krystle accompanied her mom to appointments, served as a sounding board and provided physical care when needed. Her voice of experience as a daughter serving in the support role will be featured throughout the coming chapters.

Earnestine provides the same commentary for the patient's book, *Breast Cancer Treatment Handbook*.

Brian Cluxton — Support Partner

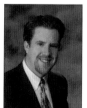

Brian was starting the phase of his life that most men look forward to—settling down with the girl of his dreams. He was getting married.

The wedding went off without a hitch. They went to Jamaica for their honeymoon. Anna, his wife, shared with him that she could feel a lump under a flat area of the skin on her breast. When they arrived home as a new couple, she called her OB/GYN who decided to perform an ultrasound and immediately decided a mammogram was also needed. She had a surgical consult with a fine needle biopsy seven days after they had been sitting on a beach in Jamaica. Twenty minutes after the biopsy, they heard the words, *"Well, it looks positive for cancer."* Brian recalls, *"We were completely flattened by the news. I can't even remember what else the doctor said to us after those words."*

One month after the wedding, Anna underwent seven hours of surgery for a mastectomy with an immediate TRAM flap reconstruction. All 16 lymph nodes removed from surgery came back negative. Anna had chemotherapy. The day of her first chemo treatment, Brian shaved his head to show his support. Looking back, he recalls, *"When other couples are starting out their new life together, I was sitting on the bathroom floor holding Anna as she was throwing up."*

Brian reflects, *"She was young—too young for breast cancer, some would think. But breast cancer does happen to young women. … Cancer has changed our lives as individuals and as a couple. Anna is the president of the Young Survival Coalition, which educates and supports young people with breast cancer. Daily she interacts with other women hearing the same words we heard—the biopsy is positive for cancer."*

Anna and Brian's life changed quickly. They were a very young couple facing a breast cancer diagnosis, but they have allowed an unexpected visitor to turn their lives into a mission to help others. I asked Brian to share how a young support partner thinks and responds to the different decisions that have to be made. Throughout this book you will read Brian's response to Anna's cancer diagnosis as a young newlywed and a support partner. Anna provides the same commentary for the patient's book, the *Breast Cancer Treatment Handbook.*

Dear Support Partner

You are reading this book because someone you care about has been diagnosed with breast cancer. You may be a spouse, sibling, child or friend who will be sharing the unfolding events of cancer treatment with someone you love. Your new role may have been decided by choice or by default. For some of you, this will be your first experience with the world of cancer treatment. For others, you may have walked this path with someone before. As you read this, you may be feeling alone in your new role. It may seem that all the rest of the world is going on their merry way while your life, and the life of the one you love, has come to a sudden stop. Cancer has changed everything.

Until you have inherited the role, the role of a caregiver is one that has little interest—now, there is a strong need to understand what to do. Whatever your situation, I wish I could sit with you and talk about what has been happening to this point and determine how I can best help you. Since that is impossible, I've written this book to talk to you as if we were talking face-to-face about your role in supporting your loved one through cancer.

So much of the information throughout the following chapters reflects my own experience of supporting people that I loved through their cancer experiences—first, my dad with acute leukemia and then, my sister-in-law with breast cancer. I added to these first-hand experiences the study of psycho-oncology (psychological, social, behavioral and ethical aspects of cancer) and working as a Breast Health Navigator with patients. As a Breast Health Navigator, I intervened with the patient and her family at the time of diagnosis and worked with them through recovery. What I learned from this is that support partners and families are often forgotten by the healthcare team. Yet, the support partner has one of the most important and pivotal roles in how a patient copes. I also learned that caregivers' worlds are disrupted and turned upside down just like the patients—in different ways of course, but causing just as much stress.

Your stress as a support partner comes from empathetically caring and supporting the patient while dealing with your own breaking heart and controlling your emotional despair in the midst of taking on a multitude of new responsibilities. Cancer is described as an emotional rollercoaster filled with uncertainty. It is much easier to deal with issues when we know how long they will last and exactly what will happen. The outcomes of cancer treatment do not come pre-packaged with results; rather, they unfold as the journey progresses.

Most often, the physical components and clinical issues of treatment are freely discussed by the healthcare team, yet the "non-physical" or emotional and social issues of living with cancer are rarely talked about. In this book, we will talk about the issues you face as a support partner and caregiver. Hopefully, discussing the "feeling" or emotional side of living with cancer on a day-to-day basis will give you the tools to remove some of the uncertainty and stress from your journey as a support partner.

As I look back over my experience of serving as a caregiver—despite all of the role changes, stresses, interruptions in my schedule, heartaches and caregiver fatigue—I can say with authority that "being there for them when it counted" far outweighed the stress of serving as their support partner. When I look back, it's clear that I was the one who was blessed.

"It sometimes takes a cross between heroism and martyrdom to survive as a primary caregiver," says Carole Levine who conducted clinical studies about the role of caregivers. During the coming days and months ahead you will surely swing between the two feelings—hero and martyr. No matter what you may be feeling, just know that the support you provide to the one you love is as helpful as any medicine she will receive.

It is my privilege to share this journey with you,

Judy

Support partners
run toward the one they love
when in need, and not away.

They feel the heartfelt pain
of the other.

They lift the other up when
they are down.

They share their fears and
tears unashamedly.

They wait and pray together when
the future is unknown.

They share the most important
gift of all, support—the ability to share
one's own heart,
even while it is breaking.

Judy Kneece

Support Partner
Perspectives

"My wife had always been the caretaker and caregiver in our family. She nursed us during illness, praised our accomplishments, encouraged us in our trials, paid the compliments, initiated the hugging—now the roles were reversed. She needed these things from me. My world had been shaken to the core. I wasn't sure I could be what she needed."

—Al Barrineau, Support Partner

"We were newlyweds. I was just learning to become a husband when I was cast into the role of support partner for my wife with breast cancer. To say I was overwhelmed in my ability to meet this new challenge was an understatement."

—Brian Cluxton, Support Partner

"I had always been a daughter who supported my mom— throughout good and bad times in our lives. But, now, there was a need for me to assume a major supporting role—she needed me in a new way; our roles were about to change."

—Krystle Brown-Shaw, Support Partner

What Is a Support Partner?

ancer is one of the most terrifying words in the English language. When you hear the word applied to someone you love, its meaning amplifies and grows to paralyzing proportions. Shock, fear, confusion and denial may absorb your mind and body after hearing the news. In the midst of the shock you are experiencing after having someone you love diagnosed with breast cancer, action must be taken. Yet, there is no "Breast Cancer 101" training to prepare you to know what to do or say, where to go for help or how to be the most supportive person to someone you love. You have inherited a new role—**support partner**—a role with many new demands and no formal training.

Your relationship to the one diagnosed may be as a spouse, significant other, sibling, child or friend. The commonality of the relationship is that the patient is someone for whom you care deeply and are committed to helping through this unknown journey of a breast cancer diagnosis. You are her support partner—a role that she did not have to recruit you for, but that you willingly volunteered for because of your deep caring and commitment to her well-being.

The Role of the Support Partner Defined

You have inherited a new role: support partner for a breast cancer patient. Some people may call you a caregiver, but your role is different from that of the medical team. Doctors and nurses work to heal the body. You work toward recovery, too, but your job also includes moral support.

What else does the role of support partner include? It is best described by the *American Heritage Dictionary* (Fourth Edition):

support v. 1. To bear the weight of, especially from below. 2. To hold in position so as to keep from falling, sinking or slipping. 3. To be capable of bearing; withstand. 4. To keep from weakening or failing; strengthen. 5. To provide for or maintain, by supplying with money or necessities. 6. To furnish corroborating evidence for. 7. To aid the cause, policy or interests of. 8. To endure; tolerate. 9. To act in a secondary or subordinate role to.

support n. 1. a. The act of supporting. b. The state of being supported. 2. One that supports. 3. Maintenance, as of a family, with the necessities of life.

partner n. 1. One that is united or associated with another or others in an activity or a sphere of common interest. a. A spouse.

A support partner is someone who helps you maintain your balance during a crisis; someone bound to you by a relationship, commitment or a common bond of interest. Support partners stand alongside the ones they love as a stabilizing force, sharing the emotional and physical burdens.

The Unexpected Challenge

As you have no doubt experienced first-hand by the time you are reading this book, a breast cancer diagnosis stresses and shakes the equilibrium of not only the patient, but those closest to her. However, the stress experienced by the support person often goes unnoticed. *"Does anyone recognize how stressful this is on my life?"* is often the unspoken thoughts of support partners as they struggle with their new role.

Why is the role of support partner so difficult? Dr. Marilyn T. Oberst, developer of the Oberst Caregiving Burden Scale, investigated the role of support partners during their loved one's cancer experience and concluded:

> *Learning to live with cancer is clearly **no** easy task. Learning to live with someone else's cancer may be **even more difficult**, precisely because no one recognizes just how hard it really is to deal with someone else's cancer.*

Yes, living with someone else's cancer is a challenge; but it is one which can be mastered successfully. The key is to learn how to manage and balance the emotional and physical demands.

Learning From the Experience of Others

The best way to learn is from others who have faced and met the challenge of filling the role of support for a breast cancer patient. Because peers can add much needed understanding and guidance, many examples quoted in this book are from other support partners.

Many patients and their support partners openly shared with me their pain and efforts to make "sense out of a senseless situation" in hopes that breast cancer support partner experiences will be more positive for those, like you, who inherit the role. I once was told, *"If you want to find your way out of a forest, it is not as helpful to ask a forester, who knows all about the trees, but to ask someone who was lost but managed to find the way out of the forest."* This book contains the experiences of those who managed to find their own way through the forest of the breast cancer experience.

It is now my desire to help you understand the challenge of living with the pain of someone else's breast cancer diagnosis, and to assist you in becoming a more effective support person. This requires a delicate balance of taking care of her needs, while you also take care of yourself.

This book is not designed as a comprehensive manual on coping. Instead, it is a combination of life experiences from patients, their support partners and my clinical experience. I urge you to reach out to other professionals— counselors, physicians, nurses and support groups—to complete your understanding of the "support" role.

Through this book you will also gain an understanding of the basics of the breast cancer treatment process. You will learn effective and supportive techniques to ease the process, and you will find additional resources available to assist you. The support role is not an easy one, but it is one from which you can learn and grow as you provide one of the most powerful tools for recovery from breast cancer—effective support.

*R*emember...

Your role as a support partner is one of the most important components for the emotional recovery of the one you love.

Support Partner
Perspectives

"When Anna went for a breast biopsy, I thought it would just be a cyst, like her mother had had. The biopsy was no big deal; besides, it was so simple it was being done as an outpatient procedure. Anna was only 32—too young for cancer. When her pathology report came back with the diagnosis of "cancer," I went into an emotional shock that lasted for days. It had never occurred to me that it would be cancer. I could not sleep at all the first few days. My mind kept torturing me with the fact that Anna could die and I would be a widower at 28."

—Brian Cluxton, Support Partner

"Shock and fear best describe my first reaction. This was only supposed to happen to other women—not my wife. We were both in a daze. But one thing was for sure; my wife and I were in this together from the start."

—Al Barrineau, Support Partner

"My mom—the strong one in my life—had been diagnosed with cancer. The thought of 'you can die from cancer' instantly flooded my mind. This thought literally tore my heart out. I could not even imagine what life would be like without her in my life. I was only 24—too young to be without her."

—Krystle Brown-Shaw, Support Partner

CHAPTER 2

The Initial Diagnosis

"You have breast cancer" are four words that forever change lives. The patient and those closest to her are suddenly faced with an unexpected challenge. Unplanned. Unprepared. Helpless. Confused. These are terms that describe the diagnostic period. Then, in the middle of all of the emotions, the patient is pressed to make critical decisions about treatment. Most patients and their support partners are ill-prepared for the decisions they are required to make concerning surgery and treatments. As previously stated, there is no "Breast Cancer 101" course to prepare for this life experience. Most are thrust into the experience without warning and forced to quickly make decisions that have lifetime effects.

If you are feeling overwhelmed, emotionally and physically, about the tasks that lay ahead of both of you, **you are normal.** Most people feel intensely ill-prepared and afraid of what the future holds. Understanding the emotions involved in a breast cancer diagnosis is as important as understanding the physical treatments. The healthcare team is prepared to take care of the physical components—surgery, radiation and chemotherapy treatments. However, most patients and their support partners are left to navigate their own way through the emotional maze in which they find themselves.

Understanding the emotional aspects of a diagnosis is essential. Understanding what you can do to manage the crisis that suddenly turns your life upside down is equally important.

Emotional Adjustment

The time from diagnosis through surgery is an acute phase of adjustment for the patient, support partner and family members. During this time, you will all be required to learn about the disease and its treatments, while dealing with all of the emotions a cancer diagnosis brings. Learning to communicate effectively with the healthcare team and the patient may also be a challenge and require new skills. Your goal is to successfully maneuver through the experience and emerge emotionally intact.

Coping Together Will Be Based On:

- Personality of the patient

- Personality of the support partner

- Previous problem solving and coping skills of the patient

- Previous problem solving and coping skills of the support partner

Even though the experience is different for the two of you, many problems and their solutions are common to not only the patient, but to you as the support person. During an unexpected crisis, there are some general physical and emotional changes that you may notice in the patient—or yourself. It is helpful to know that these symptoms are all signs of stress.

Stress Change Symptoms:

- **Body**—headaches, feelings of exhaustion, stomach problems, minor pains, decreased resistance to colds, flu, etc.

- **Mind**—negative thoughts, confusion, difficulty concentrating, sleeplessness, forgetting details, mind going blank, lower productivity

- **Feelings**—anxiety, anger, fear, frustration, emotional withdrawal

People experience these symptoms of stress in varying degrees. They are not a result of illness, but instead, they are natural, emotional reactions affecting the physical body during a crisis. Awareness of the symptoms and monitored rest are needed.

One of the most effective strategies for managing stress symptoms is support. Your support for your loved one and the support you seek for yourself will reduce the stress of the crisis. Support is a buffer against stress and a very important factor during a crisis. If reactions become severe or unmanageable for either of you, contact your healthcare provider. The medical team is available to help you, but they can only do so when you let them know your needs.

The Value of Buffering Stress

Stress, if not relieved, can take a physical toll on the body. Stress is more than just a case of "nerves" that needs to be endured; it is a physiological process that creates physical changes in the body. It is not just in your mind; it affects the entire body. Dr. Don Colbert, author of *Deadly Emotions: Understand the Mind-Body Spirit Connection That Can Heal or Destroy You,* described the wide effect of stress:

> *Stress reactions at the cellular level are pervasive and far-reaching. Fear triggers more than fourteen hundred known physical and chemical stress reactions and activates more than thirty different hormones and neurotransmitters in the body. … The body cannot differentiate between stress that physical factors cause and stress that emotional factors cause. Stress is stress. And the consequences of too much unmediated stress are the same regardless of the factors that led to a buildup.*

Too much unrelieved stress can take a physical toll on the body. It is imperative that you learn to balance your caregiving with self-care to reduce your own stress.

Acting as a support person for the patient reduces the intensity of stress she feels and, in turn, will impact her physical condition, as well as her mental condition. Your role is an invaluable one. As you stand beside her, supporting and assisting her as she deals with her diagnosis, you will be adding a component as valuable as any medicine she will receive.

*R*emember...

A crisis may cause physical as well as mental changes.

Seek the advice of your healthcare team if the symptoms become unmanageable.

Support is a valuable buffer against the stress a breast cancer diagnosis brings.

As a support partner, your supportive presence and help are as valuable as any medicine she will receive.

A Patient's Perspective on Caregivers

Ken Burger, cancer survivor and executive sports editor of *The Post and Courier*, Charleston, South Carolina, reflects on the role of his support partner during his journey with cancer:

> *The world of cancer is a parallel universe. It exists all around us. Rides with us on elevators. Parks next to us at the mall. It goes, however, mostly unnoticed. Until it becomes yours.*
>
> *A cancer diagnosis unlocks the door to this quiet, serious, sanitary world. It's the place people go to live and die with cancer. Rooms filled with faces. So many faces. You can pick out the patients. They have a certain aura. They don't talk much, but you can make them laugh. They're good company, except when they stare off into space.*
>
> *The ones you don't notice are the caregivers, God bless them. They're the ones filling out insurance forms, juggling medical bills, shuffling paperwork, chauffeuring, doing research, asking questions, making appointments, picking up prescriptions, returning calls, making choices, worrying.*
>
> *It's their job to worry. Somebody has to. Somebody has to read all the bad stuff on the Web. Somebody has to wonder what life would be like without you. Somebody has to explain it to the kids. Somebody has to imagine the unimaginable. Mostly, they're overwhelmed. But they can't show it. Or talk about it.*

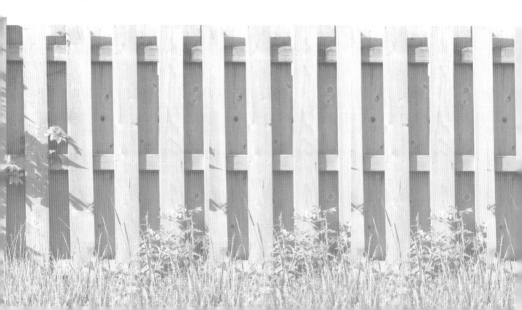

I can't say enough about the caregivers. They're an amazing breed. One thing I've seen on this unexpected journey is the need for family and friends. They're vital, but they're also vulnerable.

Far from the center of attention, their needs go unnoticed. Nerves. Nausea. Nightmares. Suffering. Silence.

For the patient, the curse of cancer comes with the blessing of an inner resolve. It kicks in right after you get the bad news. It comes over you like a notion. Something you didn't understand before suddenly seems clear. Caregivers, however, are not so blessed. From the moment of diagnosis, their world collapses into the black hole of cancer. Nothing else matters. Everything must be done. Immediately. By them. Unfortunately, cancer doesn't come with extra batteries.

While the patient sleepwalks through the netherworld of life and death, the caregiver takes out the trash, pays the exterminator, checks the homework, feeds the dog and, oh, yeah, works a full-time job, part time.

This level of concern comes at a cost—exhaustion—mentally, physically, spiritually. You see it when they're alone. The mask slips a little. The pain appears. Fear fights frustration. Shoulders slump. They are the walking wounded among us…

The ones who could use a hug, a smile, a cup of hot chocolate.

Reprinted with permission:
The Charleston Post and Courier

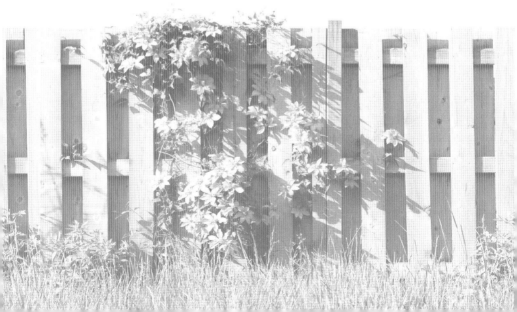

Support Partner
Perspectives

"Mom comforted me and my siblings in the days after her diagnosis. She did not want us to feel pity for her or ourselves. I should not have been surprised by her strength to deal with bad things that happen—I had seen it all my life. She had raised three children and worked two jobs to send us to school. She was still being a mom even after a cancer diagnosis, helping her children to get through this fight with minimal grief."

—Krystle Brown-Shaw, Support Partner

"My heart was broken, yet I was afraid to let Anna see me cry. I didn't want to upset her any more than she was already. However, one day my emotions became so overwhelming that I finally broke down and cried in front of her. To my surprise, it was very helpful and comforting to both of us."

—Brian Cluxton, Support Partner

"I needed to come to grips with the cancer. I thought the word cancer was an automatic death sentence. I was overwhelmed with the decisions we faced and the quick education we had to get about cancer. At the same time, I appreciated that my wife included me in the process."

—Al Barrineau, Support Partner

Dealing With Your Own Emotional Pain

*A*t the time of diagnosis, all attention from medical staff, family members and friends is directed toward the patient—naturally, because she has breast cancer. Yet, as a support partner, it is also a very difficult and painful time for you. You may be feeling overwhelmed by expectations from yourself, and others, to be strong and emotionally supportive for your loved one. You may even fear letting others see you cry as you strive to remain emotionally strong. Behind the strong facade, though, everything in your body is crying out for relief from the unexpected emotional pain. Your heart is breaking, too.

You may be surprised that you are experiencing such strong emotional reactions—after all, she is the one with cancer. It may be helpful to know that this is common for those supporting cancer patients. In fact, clinical studies by Casselith, Oberst and James discovered that spouses revealed a higher incidence of emotional problems than did the patient for up to the first 180 days after a diagnosis of cancer. This study validated the emotional challenges support partners face as they are thrust into the role of support for someone with cancer. As a support person, you, too, will find that your own emotions will need to be addressed.

It is very important for the patient's emotional recovery, as well as your own, that you recognize your pain as normal and take steps to have your own needs met. At this time, just as she needs a support network, you also need a support system to help you understand your new role as support partner.

Close emotional attachments cause support partners to suffer emotions similar to the person who is diagnosed. You may be surprised to find that you experience and mirror many of the same emotions as your partner—shock, numbness, disbelief, confusion, anger and sadness. While you may express your emotions differently because of your personality, the underlying emotions are the same.

Remember, people react differently; some people will strike out at others when angry. Others may withdraw from the person with whom they are angry. The underlying emotion is the same, even though the response is different. The important thing to remember is that you will find yourself experiencing many emotions, some of which may be new to you. For most people, dealing with a cancer diagnosis is a new experience, requiring new coping skills. It is normal to experience a wide range of emotions during the crisis created by the diagnosis. You and the patient have both been forced to embrace a dreaded enemy.

Grieving Your Loss

This is a sad time for both of you. Grieving is a natural and helpful way for healing to begin. However, many find it difficult to openly express these feelings of grief to others for fear that they may appear "weak" or "not in control." The opposite is true. These feelings show that you are very much attuned to what is occurring in your life. Expressing feelings honestly will not weaken your relationship but will strengthen it. Expressing your feelings to others helps reduce the intensity of your emotions.

Ann Kaiser Sterns summed up the scary feeling grief causes when she said, *"The experience of grief is not mental illness—it just feels that way sometimes."* At times you may feel a complete loss of control over life as you once knew it. At times you may feel as if you are "losing it" mentally. This feeling is common and is a part of working through a new life crisis.

Holding Back Emotions

Many support partners try to hold back their deep emotional pain and avoid crying in front of anyone. This is not helpful for you or the patient. Tears do not signal a "loss of control" but are more likely to convey the solidarity you feel with her. Crying is a sign that you are dealing with your emotions in a perfectly healthy and natural way. Seeing your tears will often give her the unspoken permission to share her own intense feelings and fears with you, knowing that you are very much in tune with her emotional pain.

Crying is therapeutic. After a good cry, we feel a sense of emotional release. It is similar to a rain that leaves the air clear and clean when it is over. Nicholas Wolterstroff said, *"Tears are salve on our wounds."* Gregg Levoy in *Psychology Today* shared, *"The amount of manganese stored in the body affects our moods, and the body stores 30 times as much manganese in tears as in blood serum."* Biochemist Will Frey explained, *"The lacrimal gland, which determines the flow of tears, concentrates and removes manganese from the body."* Frey has also identified three other chemicals stored up by stress that are released by crying.

If you have forced yourself to be brave and hold back your tears, now is the time to emotionally free yourself. It is okay to cry, and may even be helpful. Tears are a sign that you are in touch with reality and are dealing with the losses that a crisis brings.

Finding Your Support

As the primary support person for a cancer patient, you will find it helpful to identify someone you can talk to who understands exactly what you are feeling. This person could be a friend, family member, professional counselor or pastor. You need someone to whom you can pour out all of your fears, anxieties and emotions, knowing that you will not be judged but will be offered emotional support and guidance. It often comes as a surprise that many of the people closest to you don't understand when you try to share. They have never had to deal with what you are going through, and they feel the best way they can help is to cheer you up or help you get your mind off your problems. Being cheered up and distracted is okay, but this is not what you need now. Everyone needs at least one person to whom they can talk freely, knowing that no matter what, they will be listened to and supported.

Cancer treatment centers often offer support services, such as caregiver support groups, social workers, chaplains and counselors, who are trained to help you adjust and perform in your new role of cancer patient support. Professional counselors are skilled at crisis intervention and can identify your existing strengths and coping skills. They can help you sort out your fears and concerns and find helpful ways to face the decisions ahead. You will find that counseling professionals act as a "safe place" and allow you to say anything you think or feel without upsetting anyone.

Ask your physician, nurse or social worker for a recommendation. Remember, you need support, too. You need someone who recognizes the demands placed on a support partner and who can share this experience with you and help you master your new role. The stronger you become, the more help you can give to the patient.

Remember...

As a support partner, learning to live with someone else's cancer is difficult, but it is a task that can be mastered.

Acknowledge your own tears and emotional pain as a normal, helpful response and not as a "weakness."

Find someone you can talk to who understands your role of support partner.

It's Okay to Cry

Crying is a very acceptable and healthy expression of grief.

Crying shows how deeply you feel and how much you care.

Crying helps relieve the tension that has built up inside of you.

Crying is an expression of deep contrition and unspeakable love.

Crying speaks for you when you cannot find the words.

Crying helps you to recover your physical and emotional strength.

Crying is not the mark of weakness, but of power.

Crying allows grieving to be done in a constructive way.

Crying enables you to cope with a significant loss.

Crying is a way of communicating with your humanity.

Crying ventilates feelings of anger and hurt.

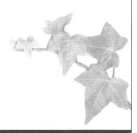

Encouragement Ministries

Support Partner
Perspectives

"Anna was the love of my life, my new bride. All I knew was that no matter what, I would be there for her. But it was important that I let her know how I viewed our future."

—Brian Cluxton, Support Partner

"Mom reacted to her diagnosis as she had to her previous life trials—strong and determined to push past the disappointment and to do what needed to be done, no matter how hard it was. Time after time, I saw her find some reason to find hope, no matter how small. That was the type of mom she had always been. Someone who thrives in tough times."

—Krystle Brown-Shaw, Support Partner

"My wife told me later that one of the best things I did to help her during those first few days was to cry with her. This seemed to really say to her, 'I'm in this with you. You are not alone.' I knew I had to put her needs first. Listening was important to her. Later, I realized this opened the door for good communication for months to come."

—Al Barrineau, Support Partner

CHAPTER 4

Understanding the Impact on the One You Love

The diagnosis of breast cancer comes unexpectedly and finds most women unprepared to deal with all of the decisions it brings. It also confirms many of a woman's greatest fears about her life and future. Facing these fears as her new reality throws her into emotional turmoil as she ponders all of the changes she must face because of cancer. Unexpected. Unprepared. Overwhelmed. Yet, no matter how she is feeling, she must move forward.

A diagnosis of breast cancer brings an array of possible losses, or threats, a woman must face. The first few days after her diagnosis, intrusive thoughts of potential losses flood her mind as she wrestles with how they could impact her future life.

Potential Losses or Threats:
- Loss or alteration of a breast
- Threat to her self-esteem because of diagnosis or surgery
- Loss or alteration of her previous feminine image
- Threat to her sexuality and attractiveness as a woman
- Threat to her future career or educational plans
- Loss of her ability to maintain her functional role in the family and/or workplace during surgery or treatments
- Concerns about her children and being unable to meet their future needs
- Threat to her life

For a short time following diagnosis, a woman most often finds herself in a state of shock, feeling mentally numb, as she sorts through the potential threats and losses. At the same time as she is struggling with these fears, she is expected to make quick, critical decisions that require a basic knowledge about her disease and treatment options.

A Patient's Greatest Loss

Diane Rice, survivor, said the hardest thing to deal with at diagnosis was *"losing control over what was happening in my life."* The most common response of a newly diagnosed breast cancer patient is the underlying theme of a "loss of control." At diagnosis, a patient has suddenly lost control over many things in her life and is faced with an unknown future filled with numerous decisions. To complicate it all, these are decisions that most people have absolutely no preparation to deal with. A breast cancer patient is forced—at a time in her life when anxieties are at their highest—to learn about breast cancer and the treatments for it.

As a support partner, you can greatly help restore her sense of control by understanding her emotional state, assisting her in a manner suitable to her personality and helping her get the information she needs to make decisions.

Creating a Safe Space for Her Emotionally

Most women react to the diagnosis of breast cancer with intense fear and emotional withdrawal. Some find it very difficult to communicate their fears and feelings at this early time. This is normal. She needs time to grieve over the diagnosis and her potential losses. Now is the time to create a "safe space" for her emotionally. Try not to be judgmental, whether you think she is responding appropriately or not. Remember, there is no right or wrong response for a woman dealing with a breast cancer diagnosis.

Dealing With Her Tears

This is also an extremely hard time for you—particularly the tears, because instinctively your desire is to "make things right" and stop her flow of tears. However, as we have previously mentioned, tears can be a necessary part of reconciling the loss. Tears are considered a normal, healthy reaction to her diagnosis. Allow her this time and space to experience her emotions in her own way. Some women cry for days or weeks—or every time they talk about their cancer—while others shed few tears, often in private.

Whatever her response, let her grieve her loss. Simply stay close by with loving support. Don't ever tell her to "stop crying because it won't help anything." This response can cause an increase in the emotional pain she is experiencing.

Dr. Susanna McMahon, Ph.D., in her book the *Portable Therapist,* discussed the topic of absence or abundance of tears during a crisis. Her unique explanation helps us understand why some people cry and others do not:

> *Too much crying or the inability to cry at all means that there is a lack of trust in ourselves and that we are trying to control our feelings. We grow up believing that giving in to our feelings is wrong and that we are weak if we do so. We cry* **too much** *when we do not trust that we can take care of ourselves. We* **never cry** *at all when we are afraid of tears. Both reflect the fear that we cannot control ourselves. When we cry all the time, we have given up and given in and feel hopeless and lost. When we never cry at all, we are also afraid—afraid of being out of control and being helpless. Both crying all the time and never crying at all are not real. Tears when we are sad or moved or very happy are as natural as blowing our noses when we have a cold. Stop hating tears—either the abundance or the lack of them. Give yourself permission to cry.*

What Most Women Want

Women have said that what they needed most immediately after their initial diagnosis was not elaborate words or deeds, but reassurance that their loved one would be with them throughout the ordeal. Their greatest need seems to be your silent presence and assurance that you will be with them through this trial. Words don't seem to be as important and are often unheard, but your close presence is remembered and appreciated. Try to give her room to grieve in the way she feels necessary without being judgmental. Don't try to tell her what to do unless she asks. Assure her of your continued commitment to the relationship. The magical words every woman wants to hear are, *"Whatever comes, I am here with you."*

Anger—A Positive Sign

During the emotionally charged period following diagnosis, your loved one may display angry outbursts. It may be the first time you have seen her angry, and you may find it difficult to understand. She may express anger toward herself for not seeking medical attention earlier or for her non-compliance with screening guidelines. She may direct her anger at the healthcare team for some reason. To your surprise, her anger may also be directed toward you. *"Why me? I am the one trying to help her,"* you may wonder. Loss and fear create anger. Anger needs a target for its expression. An easy target is someone close to her—spouse, children, parents or close friends. This display usually is not meant to be a personal attack, but is rather an effort to regain or maintain control. Often, in her mind, it is not okay to get angry with her doctors, nurses or God. Therefore, that anger may be displaced onto you or family members.

Dealing With Her Anger

View her anger as a positive sign that she is not emotionally succumbing to the diagnosis but is beginning to fight back. Forgive her, and don't view the bitterness and frustration as being directed personally toward you. Don't abandon her physically or emotionally if this occurs. This will all pass.

One woman remarked:

> *In my fit of anger and tears at diagnosis, I pushed my husband away emotionally. The one thing that happened that made a difference was a note he left reaffirming his love and the fact that this had made him more aware than ever of how important I was to him, and that he would always be here with me. This allowed me to hear what I was afraid to ask. I needed, more than anything, to be reassured that this would not cause me to lose the most important person in my life; my breast was enough to lose.*

Confirmation of your love and your continued presence are the best responses you can give during the time immediately following diagnosis. Find your own way to convey your message of commitment to her during this crisis—tell her, write her notes or show her by your actions.

Predicting How She Will Respond

Her emotional response during the entire cancer experience and the type of support she wants will be affected by her personality and prior coping skills. Women respond differently to the diagnosis and make decisions according to their personalities. Keep in mind, there is no right or wrong response. Each response originates from complex differences in personalities and is colored by life's experiences. As a support partner, your awareness of the wide range of responses and desires for support among patients will prepare you to understand that her response may not be the one you would choose, but it is her preferred choice—the right choice for her.

Emotional Response at Diagnosis

Some women may become hysterical and tearful when they hear the words, "You have breast cancer." Others may sit stoically and show very little emotion in public. For some, it will take days before they are able to talk to you about what has happened and what they are feeling; yet, for others, they want to discuss it immediately.

Information About Their Cancer

Some women want all the available facts, opinions and information they can gather; others want only the basic information needed to make a decision. Too much information can be distressing for some women; not enough information can be distressing for others.

Type of Support Desired

Some women want their support partner constantly by their side after diagnosis. Others feel a need to withdraw privately to sort through their problems on their own. Some want their partner's verbal input and opinions on treatment options. Others prefer to make their own decisions. Some want their support partner present at every office visit or treatment, and still others feel that this is too emotionally crowding and prefer to go alone unless they are physically unable.

Communication Style Preferred

Some women find it easy to communicate their emotional pain. Others find it difficult to express their feelings. This rarely changes after a cancer diagnosis. Some women speak up for what they want from you and their healthcare team, while others find this very difficult. Some patients want to tell all of their friends, while others do not want them to know the details.

Breast Conservation or Mastectomy Decision

One of the major decisions that she may have to make is between breast conservation surgery (lumpectomy) and mastectomy (removal of the entire breast). Most think that age would be the major factor impacting her choice. Age, surprisingly, is not a determining factor of a woman's decision as to the type of surgery she chooses. It is a misconception to assume that older women will not be affected by the impact of surgery as greatly as younger women and are not interested in preserving their body image. Some 75-year-old women do not want to have their breast removed and request breast-conserving surgery or immediate reconstruction. Some women in their early thirties may request a mastectomy because of their fears of recurrence or radiation therapy, thus placing very little emphasis on body image. Personal perception, not age, is what determines how women make surgical decisions.

As a support partner, be cautious about expressing strong opinions about the type of surgical procedure you think would be best. Pressure from you for one procedure or another—mastectomy or lumpectomy—can add to the patient's stress. As a support partner, it is helpful for you to learn about the options and be able to discuss them with her; however, it is necessary to allow her to make the final decision and feel she has your support for her decision. When a woman is allowed to take the lead in deciding how she wants her body image preserved or restored, she seems to adjust better to the procedure and to her new, altered body image.

Body Image After Surgery

Some women do not want to leave the hospital after a mastectomy without a temporary prosthesis to camouflage the change in their body image. For others, they do not consider this an important issue. Some women feel comfortable going without a bra after mastectomy at home and even in public, while others never want to be seen without wearing their prosthesis. We cannot predict the value a woman places on her body image. Each patient needs to decide what she feels most comfortable doing. Your job as a support partner is to support her in what she decides is best for her.

Acceptance of New Body Image

Some patients find looking at their scar area with their significant other after surgery disturbing and tend to hide to undress. Others feel very comfortable about showing their scar area and openly dress and undress. A woman will also respond to her altered body image based on the value she places on her breast and body image.

Support Is Not a Cookie-Cutter Job

As you can tell, your job as a support partner will not be a simple, cookie-cutter approach because the one you are supporting is an individual. Each area of support and assistance requires that you discover her needs. The best predictor of how she will react throughout the breast cancer experience is how she has responded to past life crises. Take this as your clue as to how she will probably respond and the basis for your support plan. If you are unsure about her needs or what she expects from you, ask specifically if a certain action will be helpful. Simply ask, *"How can I best help you with this?"* This question may prevent a lot of emotional distress for both of you by allowing her to verbalize how she wants to be supported in a decision or issue.

Remember...

A woman responds to the diagnosis of breast cancer according to her basic personality and previous coping experiences.

Her response is greatly influenced by her perception of how breast surgery will change her personal body image.

There is no right or wrong emotional response to a diagnosis.

As a support partner, you need to create a "safe space" for her to work through her emotions.

Most women desire your silent, caring presence more than elaborate words or deeds.

Angry outbursts are a sign that she is fighting back rather than succumbing to the diagnosis.

Confirmation of your love and continued support is vital, whatever her response.

Support Partner
Perspectives

"Despite all the macho training our society provides, there are some things we can't fix. My persistent urge was to make it all right, but I was forced to learn that cancer was one of those things I could not 'fix.'"

—Brian Cluxton, Support Partner

"My wife has always coped extremely well during times of crisis. She becomes very organized. She develops a plan of action and puts it into motion. She immediately seeks as much information as she can regarding the crisis. I knew this was one of the first things she needed from me—my help and support as we tried to find out about this enemy that had invaded her body."

—Al Barrineau, Support Partner

"This was my only mom. No doubt ever crossed my mind as to what I would do. I would be there for her, as she had always been for me. Helping her get through this was the most important job in my life. Helping her became my priority. Role reversal was now in order. I remember telling her 'I know you are my mom, but this time I AM helping you.'"

—Krystle Brown-Shaw, Support Partner

CHAPTER 5

What Do I Do First?

Someone you love has learned she has breast cancer. The diagnosis naturally comes as a shock to both of you. The two of you are dealing with a potentially life-threatening disease that requires proper and prompt treatment. This news automatically causes you to want to take immediate action to protect and support her. Your natural desire is to help her face treatment in any way you can. You are her front-line support in her fight to eradicate her cancer. For most, this new role of support partner for a cancer patient is one that comes unexpectedly and with no prior training—the training comes on-the-job as you take steps to help. The goal is to understand how you can be of the most help. Sometimes it may seem counter-intuitive to what you want to do. One support partner recalled:

When I heard the words 'breast cancer' from the physician, I felt I had to do everything to protect the one I loved from the hurt. I became mobilized for action. I had to do something. I became very verbal in my opinions as to what she needed to do next on the way home from the physician. The problem came when I took actions, which later I found were not needed or appropriate for her diagnosis. I learned I had added much pressure to the pain she was feeling instead of being helpful.

The Right First Step

As a support partner, you may feel compelled to act to make things better. However, in order to take the appropriate steps, it is essential to know how you can best help. The first guideline is knowing that you must allow her time to come to grips with the emotional impact.

Assess what you can do that will be most helpful to her. Remember, the question, *"How can I be most helpful to you at this time?"* may prevent many problems by offering the kind of support she really wants and needs.

The patient has had no preparation to deal with all of the emotions and complex decision-making demands that accompany the diagnosis. At diagnosis, when she feels overwhelmed, you may be most helpful by locating sources of information specific to her diagnosis. Becoming knowledgable about her cancer is necessary.

The Power of Knowledge

Knowledge about a subject implies mastery, yet it also acknowledges reality. As a support partner you want to know as much as possible about her illness, yet you may be fearful about what you will learn. Think of learning about her cancer as a means of being better equipped to help her. Facing your own fears of understanding what her diagnosis encompasses is the beginning of preparing yourself to better help her. There will be many stressful decisions and events she will need to face. Understanding what is ahead will allow you to anticipate the event and help her understand, which will take some of the trauma out of a stressful event. Stress is better managed when it is anticipated.

The best source for accurate information about her cancer is from her treatment team. With the emergence of the Internet, it is an easy place to go to for information; however, it can be a source of inappropriate information for her cancer. Limit your searches to recognized authorities such as the National Cancer Institute (NCI) and the American Cancer Society. Ask your treatment team for information on her cancer and treatment. Identify someone on the treatment team with whom you can comfortably communicate and who can provide or recommend additional resources appropriate for her cancer when needed. The overwhelming desire to "make things better" needs to be directed with correct information. Take time to learn the basics of her disease, treatment options, what steps need to be taken and in what time frame.

Cancer Treatment Decisions

Very seldom is breast cancer a medical emergency (an exception is inflammatory breast cancer, which requires immediate treatment). Most women have several weeks to learn about their disease and consider various treatment options before submitting to surgery, chemotherapy or radiation treatments. In most cases, breast cancer has been in a woman's body for years. A tumor that has a normal growing cycle (doubles every 100 days) and is one centimeter in size (⅜ inch, the size of the tip of a woman's smallest finger) could have been in her body for eight or more years and has just now become detectable. (See graphic on page 53.) Several more weeks in which to gather information and make educated, appropriate decisions will not adversely affect the outcome for the patient.

Several weeks is a short period of time; therefore, your assistance in finding the right information will facilitate helping her work as an informed patient with her treatment team in making treatment decisions. Women who receive support while reviewing their options, without pressure on specifics from their support partner, will have the foundation needed for emotional recovery.

Remember...

Allow her time to absorb the emotional impact.

Obtain correct information from your treatment team before surging ahead with advice or decision making.

Assess how you can best help; resist the urge to rush the patient or to insist on any particular treatment option.

Support Partner
Perspectives

"Surprisingly, I was the child in the picture after Mom's diagnosis. I was blessed with her interactions and communications with me. There were no charades; Mom was always open and honest with me about all the details of her cancer. This made it easier for me to deal with our new relationship."

—Krystle Brown-Shaw, Support Partner

"Being open and honest with our children helped us all. My wife had always been there for us. Now it was time for us to be her support and strength. Taking care of Mom helped the boys to deal with their emotions."

—Al Barrineau, Support Partner

CHAPTER 6

Telling the Children

If children are included in the circle of the diagnosis of cancer, the most common question is, *"What do we tell the children?"* The best answer is, *"The truth!"* Children are very perceptive. They know and sense much more than they could ever communicate. They will immediately feel that something is wrong in the family, even if you decide not to tell them. What they imagine may be much worse than the truth. From the beginning, it is imperative that there is openness and honesty with them about what is occurring in the family.

They need to hear the truth from someone they trust, using a language level they can understand. You do not have to tell everything that is happening, but you need to give them enough information so they will not feel excluded. Finding out from someone outside of the family can weaken a child's trust, resulting in a lowered trust factor in the future.

Impact of Diagnosis on Children

Families often worry about the effect the illness will have on their children. The most important factor in how they respond is how they see the family respond to the illness. If they see you communicating openly and honestly while sharing with a positive attitude, they will be more likely to respond the same way. The family can value this time as one of growth and maturity in problem solving. If you find it difficult to know what to say, or if you realize problems are developing in the family with the children, contact your cancer treatment center and ask for a reference for a counselor trained in dealing with children.

The diagnosis of cancer in a family is an unwanted event; however, it can serve as an opportunity for personal growth, even in children. David Pertz, M.D., in his book, *How Do We Tell the Children?*, explains:

> *A child's first question about illness and death is an attempt to gain mastery over frightening images of abandonment, separation, loneliness, pain and bodily damage. If we err on the side of overprotecting them from emotional pain and grief with 'kind lies,' we risk weakening their coping capacities.*

Tips for Telling the Children:

- If possible, wait until there is some emotional control in communication. For some, this may take a day or two; others may be able to share the first day.

- Ask the treatment team for information, or call the local American Cancer Society for information written for children about a loved one's cancer.

- Plan what you will say to the children and find a time and place when the conversation will not be interrupted. Turn off the television and the telephone to prevent interruptions.

- Start by sharing something similar to the following: *"Mommy* (or name called) *has found a lump in her breast. The doctor says that the lump is cancer* (call it by the right name). *Cancer cells grow very fast. The doctors say that they need to take this lump out because these are not good cells. The doctors and nurses can also help by giving medicine."*

- Continue to share truthfully and simply what the facts are. If you have an example that will help explain, such as their experience of getting medicine from a doctor to help them feel better when they were ill, this will be helpful.

- Young children's greatest concern is often about themselves—*"Who will take care of me?", "Where will I stay?"*

- Assure the children that their thoughts and actions did not cause the cancer and that they cannot catch the cancer.

- If anyone begins to cry, assure the children that this is because they are sad and it is okay to express feelings by crying.

- Allow the children to ask questions. Answer to the best of your ability. If you do not know the answers, be honest and say you do not know. Keep your answers age-appropriate.

- Reassure them that you will continue to tell them what is happening.

- Involve them in the process of helping Mom adjust to surgery and possible treatments. Help them to feel as if they are part of the solution to the problem by sharing chores that contribute to the well-being of the family.

- Similar to adults, teens will respond according to their personalities— some are very emotional and some are very reserved in their demeanor. Teens are in the life developmental stage of breaking away, so don't be surprised if they don't seem to be overly concerned and quickly return to their normal duties and interests. Take this as a compliment; your openness has restored their confidence that, as a family, you can cope with your new situation.

Telling the Teachers

It is suggested that you tell the teachers or instructors of your children that your child is dealing with a cancer diagnosis (or family crisis) at home. This alerts them and allows them to identify potential changes in a child's behavior as stress reactions to the change in their home environment. This knowledge allows them to offer support and understanding, rather than correction, if a child should act out. They will also be able to recognize if the child is suffering from overwhelming sadness and needs emotional support. Older children and teens may feel more comfortable sharing their feelings with adults outside of the home rather than with their parents.

Teachers are also often in a position to request help and assistance from other school personnel, such as trained professional counselors and school psychologists, in order to offer additional professional emotional support to a child.

When to Seek Professional Help:

- Marked change in school performance

- Poor grades despite trying very hard

- Extreme worry or anxiety manifested by refusing to go to school, go to sleep or take part in age-appropriate activities

- Frequent angry outbursts or anger expressed in destructive ways

- Hyperactive activities, fidgeting, constant movement beyond regular or normal behaviors

- Persistent anxiety or phobias

- Accident proneness or self-punishment
- Persistent nightmares or sleeping disorders
- Stealing, promiscuity, vandalism, illegal behavior (drug/alcohol use)
- Persistent disobedience or aggression (longer than six months) and violations of the rights of others
- Opposition to authority figures

Children's Support Resource

Kids Konnected (www.kidskonnected.org) is an organization committed to supporting children involved in a family cancer diagnosis. For the cost of postage (approximately $6.95), they will send care packages to children. Packages are tailored to each family depending on the age of the children, who has cancer and in what stage it is diagnosed. Packages contain books, workbooks, brochures and additional information to help the child or teen better cope with the changes cancer brings. Every package includes a "Hope" teddy bear for each child and a security blanket for children under five.

*R*emember...

Children need to be told the truth by someone they trust.

An illness need not adversely affect children.

Children usually respond in a manner similar to the way they observe the adults responding.

Inform teachers and instructors of the diagnosis so they can offer additional understanding and support.

A crisis can serve as a time of growth and emotional maturity in a family unit.

Family Hardship

Part of the reality of life is hardship.
That is not a negative statement.
It is simply a statement of fact.

Every day brings new challenges.
Living with the expectation that
life will be difficult makes
hard times easier to deal with.

When a family encounters
hard times, they will need to join
together and face the challenge
as a team. They will need to be
sensitive to the needs of individual
family members, each of whom
will face unique difficulties.

Life is not easy,
but having a support system
makes life that much easier.

Family Friend Poems

37

Support Partner
Perspectives

"When it came to the bills that come with a cancer diagnosis, my attitude was, 'Who cares? Get the needed treatment, no matter what, and we will worry about the bills when they arrive.' Anna needed to know that no price was too great to pay for her future health."

—**Brian Cluxton, Support Partner**

"Being properly insured relieved us of one of the biggest problems a lot of people face—the financial responsibility of dealing with a serious illness. We were fortunate. But even if we had no insurance coverage, I would not have let that keep us from getting the medical attention my wife needed. Outstanding bills would have been a small price to pay for her life."

—**Al Barrineau, Support Partner**

"Mom worked in a hospital and knew all the 'ins and outs' about insurance. This was helpful for both of us. However, like many people, insurance was not adequate to cover all of the charges for her treatment. We had been through tough times as a family before and knew that somehow we would make it again. We had to concentrate on treatment—the paying of hospital bills would have to come later."

—**Krystle Brown-Shaw, Support Partner**

CHAPTER 7

Health Insurance and Employment Issues

W hile dealing with the emotionally overwhelming issues of breast cancer treatment, it can be equally overwhelming to cope with the financial changes incurred by a diagnosis of cancer. Bills will come from the hospital, physicians, pharmacies, treatment centers, etc. Most patients have some form of health insurance coverage to help with the medical expenses. The challenge is keeping accurate records to ensure optimal reimbursement of claims. This often means constant communication between the insurance carrier and those billing for services. As a support partner, you can play a vital role by organizing the record keeping, thereby reducing the stress brought on the patient by the barrage of bills and claims. If the patient is insured at the time of diagnosis, call the insurance provider or carefully read your policy for guidelines.

Insurance Coverage Guideline Questions:
- Requirements and procedures for pre-approval for hospital admissions
- Requirements for second opinions for surgery or treatments
- Guidelines for second opinions from physicians
- Procedure for filing claims
- Name of person at the insurance company who will handle your claims
- Amount of deductibles, if any, before claims are paid
- Limits imposed on amounts paid for surgery, chemotherapy, radiation therapy or reconstructive surgery
- Coverage for new or experimental treatments, or for clinical trials. Ask what they cover and if there are limits on amounts for such procedures.

Record Keeping

Keeping up with the filing of claims and payments can become burdensome. However, accurate record keeping and careful scrutiny of all bills make the task much simpler.

Record-Keeping Tips:

- Purchase a pocket calendar to record all appointments (decide if you or the patient will keep the calendar).

- Write on the calendar: physician visits, procedures performed, medications administered or supplies used.

- At the time of service, ask for a copy of all charges or ask to have one mailed to you.

- Keep copies of all charges for appointments, services, medications or medical supplies in one place (a designated box, file folder or drawer will serve this purpose).

- Check periodically to see if appropriate payments are being made to medical providers.

- If problems arise with payments, contact your healthcare facility or provider and ask for help in providing the information needed to receive adequate payment.

- Call your insurance provider and talk with your claims representative to offer additional records or assistance for getting information from your medical providers. (Always record the name of the person to whom you speak. You may need the name for future reference.)

- Keep all premiums current. Do not allow your insurance to lapse from lack of payment.

Insurance coverage is more difficult to obtain after any major illness. For this reason, be very careful to keep all premiums current. Before changing jobs, be certain insurance coverage is available under the new employer's benefits program. Some policies may not cover a pre-existing condition or illness.

If, for some reason, employment linked to insurance coverage is terminated, ask about COBRA (Consolidated Omnibus Budget Reconciliation Act 1986) health insurance coverage. This insurance allows certain former employees, retirees, spouses, former spouses and dependent children the right to temporary continuation of health coverage at group rates. This policy is only available when coverage is lost due to certain, specific events. COBRA is usually more expensive than health coverage for active employees; however, it is ordinarily less expensive than individual health coverage.

Financial Needs

If you realize treatment is going to be a financial burden to your family, or if you are uninsured, ask to speak to the social worker in the cancer treatment center as soon as possible. Social workers are trained to help with the social issues of the illness, including helping to secure financial help for medical services, if needed. There are various services available for cancer patients. The earlier you can make this need known, the more effective the social work team can be in helping you. Applying for help often requires filing forms and a period of waiting for approval. People often feel embarrassed to ask for help and postpone the issue. However, many people find that an unexpected illness drains their financial reserves. You are not alone. Ask for help early.

Employment Issues

A woman in treatment for breast cancer will be away from her job for some period of time, which varies among patients. Surgery can result in an absence of three to six weeks, depending on the type of surgery, healing time and the nature of her employment. Her surgeon will estimate when she will be able to return to work. Her supervisor needs to be informed of the expected sick leave time that will be necessary following surgery and/or treatment. If treatment is required after surgery, additional time away from work may be needed since chemotherapy and radiation side effects vary in patients. Ask her oncologist how much time away from work can reasonably be expected. Some women are able to work a normal schedule during treatments. Others have to curtail their activities because of treatment, taking sick leave for the treatment period. A woman's physical and emotional demands at work, plus the type of drugs in her treatment plan and her general health, will determine if she can continue to work. Only her treatment team can provide an accurate estimate of time needed for recovery.

Workplace Discrimination

Occasionally, a cancer patient may be discriminated against at her workplace because of illness; however, there are both federal and state laws to protect her. The social worker at the cancer treatment center will be able to help you in this matter.

Telling Fellow Employees and Friends

Ask the patient what information she wants her co-workers and concerned friends to know about her diagnosis and treatment. Some women are very open and talk freely about their disease and its treatment. Other women feel that their illness is private and prefer to keep the details to themselves. Knowing her wishes is helpful when friends and co-workers come to visit and call to ask about the patient. Being aware of what she wants others to know allows you to answer their questions without invading her privacy. Some women feel it is helpful if someone else communicates with the office during their illness, especially during the acute diagnostic period. Patients soon tire of "telling their illness story" and find it a relief to have someone else perform this role.

Online Communication

A solution for communications during breast cancer treatment is found on a Web site service call CaringBridge®. It offers anyone going through a health crisis a free online communication page. A health update or message can be posted at anytime. Friends and family can communicate by leaving a message that can be accessed and answered at the patient's convenience. Setting up the communication hub at www.caringbridge.org is simple and free.

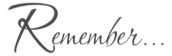*emember...*

Wise planning and record keeping can remove most of the hassle from insurance reimbursements.

Support partners can alleviate stress for the patient by performing record-keeping tasks.

Keep all insurance premiums current.

If you need financial help, ask a social worker at your cancer treatment center as early as possible.

Time away from work varies with different types of treatment. Physicians can help predict time needed for sick leave.

Issues of discrimination in employment can be brought to the attention of professionals in the area of protection for cancer patients.

Ask the patient how much information she would like her friends or co-workers to know about her illness.

Support Partner Perspectives

"Getting involved in a support group for support partners of breast cancer patients provided a haven for me. I had felt a need to be the strong one for my wife. The support group gave me the opportunity and place to express my concerns, ask my questions and voice my fears. I was with others who could truly relate to the way I felt—people who really understood."

—Al Barrineau, Support Partner

CHAPTER 8

Support Groups

*Y*ou may find that while you are providing the vital role of support for the one you love, it may be hard to reach out to others to receive your own support. The role of supporting someone through cancer treatments, with all of its many demands, is physically and emotionally exhausting and often goes unrecognized by others for the day-to-day stress it brings. Somehow, it seems okay if a patient complains about the stress and burdens treatment brings and her desire for it all to come to an end. Support partners, however, find expressing their caregiver fatigue to others as somehow unthinkable and offensive. So, support partners hunker down and continue, day after day, suffering from caregiver exhaustion in silence. You may even question if anyone would possibly understand your needs if you did reach out.

If you can relate to these feelings, know that there are many people who have walked this path of cancer patient support and understand your role with its many demands. People who understand your plight and can offer understanding advice on how to cope are found in cancer center support groups and support programs. Most cancer programs offer referrals to professionals who are available to talk, and most centers sponsor support groups for caregivers.

At a caregivers' support group, you will find others struggling with the same problems of dealing with the daily role of being emotionally "up" and supportive for someone they love, while dealing with their own physical exhaustion. Along with the exhaustion, there are fears of *"What about tomorrow?", "Is treatment working?"* and *"Are we going to beat this thing?"* Questions that are unspoken, yet they are questions that you daily contemplate. Questions which can grip your heart with fear at times when you think about possible negative outcomes.

If you are dealing with these fears in silence, support would be very beneficial for you. You find solace when another caregiver confirms that you are not inadequate or weak, but are dealing with the same physical and emotional challenges they face. Along with this comfort, you may find many tips that make your role easier. Even though you may feel you have enough support already, or cannot relate to a support group, I highly encourage reaching out to a support group or professional counselor. Many find that a support group is one of the most effective methods for emotional management.

Support groups that are disease-specific, such as one for breast cancer patients, are composed of people who are going through the same problems of learning to live life under similar circumstances. Groups are a place where people with similar fears and needs can meet to share and reduce their anguish and confusion. They are places where all anxieties, anger and apprehension are understood without any raised eyebrows as to their significance. They are also a place where you can increase your knowledge and perception of the disease that the patient is battling. Families and friends are wonderful sources of support, but only someone going through the same life crisis can fully comprehend and empathize. That's the role of support groups.

Studies have proven that, for patients, participating in support groups improves the quality of life and relationships: *"Sometimes fear is so engulfing, it precludes the ability to call for help,"* explains one patient. *"It is this fear that those of us called patients understand and can help to diminish for one another,"* writes Robert Fisher, a member of the Patient to Patient Volunteer Program. Finding a group for your loved one and one for yourself will add a new dimension to your breast cancer experience.

Look for a support group that is led by a professional facilitator who is trained in group dynamics and knows how to keep the meeting meaningful to those present. A group should offer an opportunity to share experiences, but should not be dominated by "poor me" stories. Instead, educational and support techniques should be provided at each meeting. You may want to talk with the facilitator before attending a meeting to determine whether the characteristics of the particular group meet your needs.

For information on breast cancer support groups, contact your cancer treatment center, local American Cancer Society or Young Survival Coalition Web site for a list of groups. Online support groups and blogs are also available.

*R*emember...

For many, support groups offer a safe place to express feelings and receive support.

Look for a support group that has an educational component as part of the meeting.

Support Partner
Perspectives

"*Somehow I thought that if I learned enough about breast cancer and all its treatments, we could beat it with knowledge. I was on a mission; I read tons of books and surfed the Internet, looking for the magical answer. However, I soon found that the Internet could be a very scary place for support partners of the newly diagnosed. There is a lot of misinformation out there, so stick to recommended sources of help.*"

—Brian Cluxton, Support Partner

"*We were shocked and overwhelmed by what we needed to know and what we didn't know about breast cancer.*"

—Al Barrineau, Support Partner

"*Before Mom's diagnosis, I had read about breast cancer, but that was all. I had never experienced someone close to me being diagnosed with breast cancer. This was all new to me. I did, however, know that you can die from it— one of the most terrifying thoughts I have ever had. We both learned about breast cancer quickly. It was 'on-the-job' training for both of us. We were forced to learn about breast cancer so we could do all we could to make wise decisions about her treatments and future life.*"

—Krystle Brown-Shaw, Support Partner

CHAPTER 9

Understanding Breast Cancer

Breast cancer is a very complex disease with many variables involved in its treatment. The language and terminology used by the medical profession is often unique to the disease. This chapter is designed to clarify and explain the basic facts of breast cancer in the simplest way.

The female breast is a very complicated glandular organ and is the site of the most common cancer in women—breast cancer. No one knows exactly what causes breast cancer. Genetics (having a family history of breast cancer) increases the risk. Factors that do not cause cancer, but may promote it, include lifestyle factors such as diet and hormonal function.

Cancer begins when normal cells in the breast change into cells that have an uncontrolled growth pattern. If not removed, the cancer cells continue to divide and grow and may spread to other parts of the breast and then to other parts of the body. The cancer cells can invade neighboring tissues and spread throughout the body, establishing new growths at distant sites; this process is called metastasis.

Most people think that all breast cancers are the same. However, there are approximately 15 different identified types of breast cancer. Cancers that develop from different types of breast tissue in different parts of the breast may have varying characteristics. The term carcinoma is used by physicians to describe a malignant or cancerous growth.

Internal Structure of the Female Breast

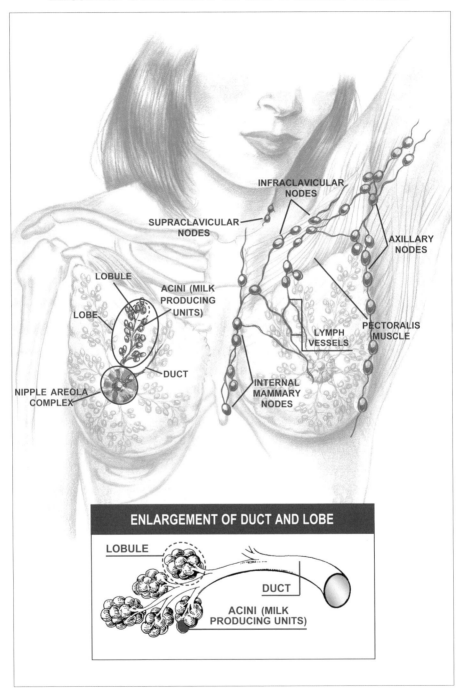

INFRACLAVICULAR NODES

SUPRACLAVICULAR NODES

AXILLARY NODES

LOBULE

ACINI (MILK PRODUCING UNITS)

LOBE

PECTORALIS MUSCLE

LYMPH VESSELS

DUCT

NIPPLE AREOLA COMPLEX

INTERNAL MAMMARY NODES

ENLARGEMENT OF DUCT AND LOBE

LOBULE

DUCT

ACINI (MILK PRODUCING UNITS)

Types of Cancers

Cancers are first classified according to their relationship to walls of their origin. The two major divisions are in situ and invasive/infiltrating.

DUCT WITH NORMAL CELLS

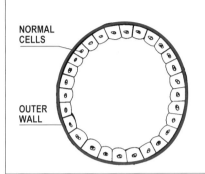

Normal ducts and lobules are lined with one or more layers of orderly cells.

IN SITU CANCER CELLS

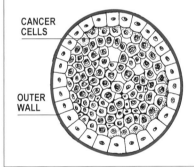

In situ carcinomas are cancers that are still contained within the walls of the portion of the breast in which they developed. The cancer has not grown through the outer wall and invaded surrounding tissue.

INVASIVE CANCER CELLS

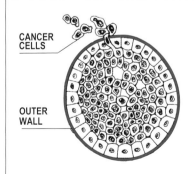

Infiltrating or **invasive carcinomas** are cancers that have grown through the duct or lobular walls and into surrounding connective tissues.

Descriptions of Cancers

Breast cancers are named according to the part of the breast in which they develop.

DUCTAL CARCINOMA	LOBULAR CARCINOMA

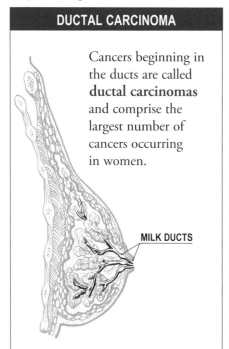

Cancers beginning in the ducts are called **ductal carcinomas** and comprise the largest number of cancers occurring in women.

MILK DUCTS

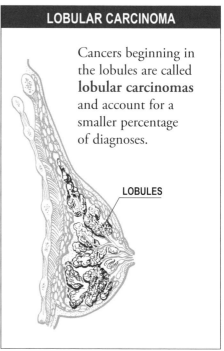

Cancers beginning in the lobules are called **lobular carcinomas** and account for a smaller percentage of diagnoses.

LOBULES

INVASIVE AND IN SITU CANCERS

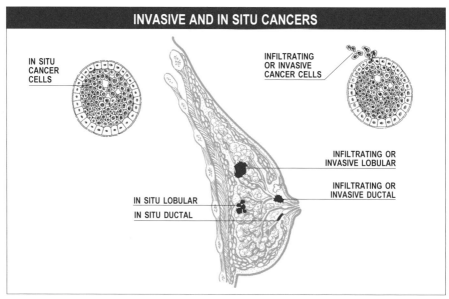

IN SITU CANCER CELLS

INFILTRATING OR INVASIVE CANCER CELLS

INFILTRATING OR INVASIVE LOBULAR

INFILTRATING OR INVASIVE DUCTAL

IN SITU LOBULAR

IN SITU DUCTAL

Growth of Breast Cancer

Some breast cancers grow rapidly, while others grow very slowly. Breast cancers have been shown to double in size every 23 to 209 days. A tumor that doubles every 100 days (an estimated average doubling time) has been in a woman's body approximately eight to ten years when it reaches one centimeter in size (⅜ inch), which is the size of the tip of her smallest finger. The cancer begins with one damaged cell and doubles until it is detected on a mammogram, by finding a lump or from symptoms such as a discharge or a change in the breast.

Some experts believe that cancers may grow in spurts and the doubling time may vary. However, when a one-centimeter tumor is found, the tumor has already grown from one cell to approximately 100 billion cells.

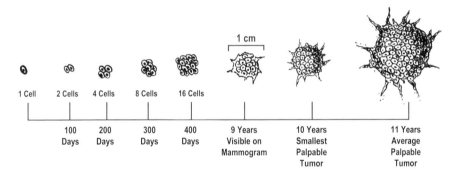

1 Cell	2 Cells	4 Cells	8 Cells	16 Cells	1 cm		
	100 Days	200 Days	300 Days	400 Days	9 Years Visible on Mammogram	10 Years Smallest Palpable Tumor	11 Years Average Palpable Tumor

Breast cancer is not a sudden occurrence; it is a process that has been developing for a period of time. Therefore, when a biopsy confirms a cancerous breast tumor, the patient is usually not facing a medical emergency. She has time to get answers to questions and learn about her particular disease and treatment options. Most physicians recommend surgery within several weeks of the biopsy. There are exceptions, such as inflammatory carcinoma (cancer in the lymphatic system), which requires immediate treatment with chemotherapy for maximum control. Ask the physician what recommendations will be made regarding the patient's particular tumor. Tests performed on the tumor will reveal cell type and estimate whether the tumor is growing slowly or rapidly.

Some tumors will have the characteristic of spreading quickly to other parts of the body. Others do not seem to spread as readily. Breast cancer spreads to other parts of the body through the lymphatic system or the blood system. The spread of the cancer can be local (in the area of the breast), regional (in the nodes or area near the breast) or distant (to other organs of the body). These characteristics will be presented in the pathology report after surgery.

Treatment Options

After a biopsy confirming cancer, a woman will usually have to make some decisions about treatment options. These decisions will include surgical procedures, and possibly radiation therapy, chemotherapy or hormonal therapy. Surgical decisions will be based on the preliminary (biopsy) study of the tumor.

When the final (surgical) pathology report is evaluated, the oncologist will decide which treatments are most appropriate for the patient's type of cancer. For some cancers, surgery may be the only treatment needed. Others may require additional treatment with radiation therapy, chemotherapy or hormonal therapy.

*R*emember...

Breast cancer is usually not a medical emergency. The patient has time to get the answers to her questions before final treatment is selected.

The biopsy pathology report is used to make surgical decisions.

The final pathology report is used to determine treatment with chemotherapy, radiation or hormonal therapy.

Silent Presence

Speaking to those who were
serving as cancer support
partners, Dr. David Spiegel
reworded the old admonition,
**"Don't just stand there,
do something,"**
to become,
*"Don't just do something,
stand there."*

Sometimes the greatest gift
we can give is our silent presence.
At times, there are no
"good" words that can be said.
The patient just needs us to stand
along beside her and silently
share her sorrow.

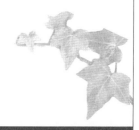

Dr. David Spiegel

Support Partner
Perspectives

"Anna had wonderful doctors she trusted, but we still felt safer having a second opinion. It helped her feel safe proceeding with recommended treatments. We shop for cars, so why not feel comfortable shopping for the best doctors and treatment options?"

—Brian Cluxton, Support Partner

"Working in a hospital proved to be helpful to Mom after her diagnosis. Because of this, she knew a lot of people. She had a great relationship with her doctors and trusted them. She listened closely to their recommendations, but we always discussed them. Sometimes we didn't agree, and sometimes we simply did not understand 'why' something was being recommended. Just listening, which my mom sometimes felt was no help at all, helped me sort out her questions and concerns, helping make her final decisions with more confidence."

—Krystle Brown-Shaw, Support Partner

"The best thing our doctors did to help us in the beginning was to keep our primary physician informed. He was the one I looked to, the one I relied on. Their cooperation and good communication were invaluable during our decision-making processes."

—Al Barrineau, Support Partner

CHAPTER **10**

Breast Cancer Decisions

any women say that after they heard the word "cancer," they remembered very little about what was discussed during the remainder of the physician's visit. However, it is essential that information about the extent of the disease and treatment options provided in this first meeting be accurately understood. Treatment decisions and the necessary steps of actions that need to be taken are dependent upon a complete understanding of what was said by her physician. If you were present, this will help in recalling the facts presented. Discuss what the physician said so that you both can be reassured and have a clear understanding of the decisions that need to be made.

If you were also overwhelmed and do not have reliable recall, clarification of information from the physician is necessary. Call her physician to schedule a return visit. It is vital to have this information before treatment options can be explored. Sometimes a period of time, usually overnight, may need to pass in order for questions to surface that need to be answered. Often the physician's nurse will be able to answer many of the general questions.

If a return call or visit is necessary, be prepared to ask all of the questions that have emerged during your discussions. Take notes or tape-record (ask permission) the answers. You may want to continue the practice of note taking or recording her consultations with the physician or nurse. In addition, ask for written information on breast cancer options for surgery and treatment recommendations following surgery. Becoming informed partners with the healthcare team is essential in order to regain a sense of control.

Most women eagerly seek help from their support partners in gathering information. Some, however, do not want any assistance past the information gathering stage. They prefer to make treatment decisions completely on their own. Therefore, communication between the two of you about the desired level of participation is crucial if your support is to be helpful to the patient.

The Decision-Making Process

There will be many decisions and conversations with the patient's healthcare team. Therefore, it will be helpful if you begin to read and acquire a basic understanding of the terminology and types of treatments. A patient's anxiety level may be so high during the diagnostic period that she cannot concentrate enough to participate in the search for information, or comprehend what she reads or hears. This will improve as time goes by. Included at the back of this book is a glossary of basic terms used in the diagnosis and treatment of breast cancer. It will be helpful to familiarize yourself with these terms.

It is very important that the information you collect is specific to the patient's diagnosis. There are approximately 15 types of breast cancer. Furthermore, treatments can vary even when women are diagnosed with the same type of cancer. Many factors are considered when developing a treatment plan. Ask her physician for the specifics of the diagnosis. Remember, her healthcare team should always be the primary source of information. There are some important questions regarding the specifics of her initial diagnosis that are helpful to ask.

Immediate Decision Questions to Ask the Healthcare Team:

- What is the name of her cancer?
- Do you have written information on her specific cancer?
- Is the cancer in situ (inside of the duct or lobular walls) or invasive (grown through the duct or lobular walls)?
- What is the size of the tumor?
- Is there any suspected lymph node involvement?
- Is cancer suspected in any other area of the same breast or the opposite breast?
- Is there evidence that the cancer has spread outside the breast and nodes?
- Where can we get written information on treatment options?

- What decisions does she need to make about her upcoming treatment? (Surgery is usually the first decision. Lumpectomy versus mastectomy; if mastectomy, reconstruction immediate or delayed. Other decisions are made after the final pathology report is available).

- In what time frame do you recommend that the decisions be made?

- Who on the healthcare team can answer our questions?

- When and how can we contact this person for questions or information? (Telephone, personal appointments, e-mail, etc.)

- Are there any characteristics about her cancer that could impact our decision making?

- Will her case be presented to a multidisciplinary conference for evaluation by a team of physicians? (Breast centers usually have conferences before surgery and treatment. A team of physicians from all disciplines review the case as a group and offer suggestions to her physicians for treatment options. This conference is usually without charge and is offered as a service to the patient.)

- If she desires a second opinion, what should be done to arrange one?

How Treatment Decisions Are Made

Physicians make treatment decisions based on more than the type of breast cancer.

Treatment Decisions Are Based On:

- The stage of the cancer (Stage 0 – 4; determined by size and how much it has spread to other parts of the body)

- Cancer receptor status for estrogen/progesterone and HER2 (determined by pathologist)

- Age and menopausal status

- General health

- Treatment goals of the patient

Before anyone can give accurate information on suggested treatment, these basic facts need to be known. Without access to the mammography film and/or report and a final biopsy pathology report describing all aspects of the tumor, any information about the patient's particular case can only be an educated guess.

The media—including television, radio and magazines—have taken up the cause of breast cancer education. However, much of this information is very general and may not apply to her diagnosis. Media information may include non-approved treatments or discoveries unavailable for public use. Also, be careful of well-meaning friends and their advice. Unless they are professionals in the field of breast cancer and have access to the pathology report, they may offer information that is not applicable and may only confuse you. Remember, the healthcare team is your best source for accurate advice based on the patient's specific diagnosis and her health status.

For more information or clarification on any of the information either of you read, call the physician's office, cancer treatment center or organizations specializing in cancer. Sources for free information are available from various professional organizations. (Names and addresses of these organizations are listed in the back of this book.)

One of the most helpful booklets on treatment decisions is *Breast Cancer: Treatment Guidelines for Patients*, produced by the National Comprehensive Cancer Network (NCCN). It provides patients, and the general public, with up-to-date information on breast cancer treatment. The NCCN Breast Cancer Treatment Guidelines are found on their Web site (www.nccn.org). The information is a consensus of recommended treatments from 19 comprehensive cancer treatment centers. These guidelines should only serve as a resource for understanding treatment options for each stage of breast cancer. Each patient must be individually evaluated. Discuss the guidelines, or other information, with the patient's physician.

Second Opinions

When a medical diagnosis is serious and the suggested therapy is difficult to accept, some women feel the need for additional information or a second opinion. Surgery, chemotherapy and radiation therapy deserve serious consideration, and the patient needs all of the information necessary to make an informed decision. A second opinion is obtained from another physician practicing in the same area of medicine. The physician reviews the patient's records and offers treatment advice. This opinion may help her feel sure about the final treatment decision. However, for some women, a second opinion may cause anxiety and increased confusion.

Some insurance providers may require a second opinion before treatment. Check with the insurance provider on this point. Physicians may refer patients for second opinions in order to validate treatment decisions. It is necessary that the patient evaluate her own needs and decide if a second opinion would be of assistance or not.

Reasons For a Second Opinion:

- She feels insecure or unsure about what she has been told about surgery or treatments.
- Insurance provider requires a second opinion.
- There has been disagreement or confusion about the right course of action.
- Patient desires information about newer therapies not offered by her treatment team.

How to Obtain a Second Opinion

If the patient feels a second opinion would help resolve her indecisiveness, ask the treatment team for names of several physicians qualified in this area. Ask the treatment team to list the pros and cons of each one in order to help determine who will best suit her needs. You may also call a major cancer treatment center for a self-referral. Some of the national cancer organizations listed in the reference section of this book will give the names of the major cancer treatment centers located in your area and the services they provide.

Second opinions are often provided through the pretreatment multidisciplinary conferences held at some centers. Physicians from all areas of breast care (radiology, pathology, surgery, medical oncology, radiation oncology, reconstructive surgery) look at the patient's records as a group, discuss her individual case, share their opinions with the group and make treatment recommendations as a team. All of this is done before any of the final treatment decisions are made. These conference recommendations serve as a guide for her own physicians to consider. If she has access to this type of conference, or a group of physicians practicing as a team, it serves as an excellent way not only to get a second opinion, but several expert opinions.

Preparing for the Second Opinion Visit

When seeking a second opinion, the goal is to clarify any questions. Make a list of questions and concerns before the visit and take the list to the appointment. Also, be sure that all requested lab and diagnostic test results are sent to the physician before her visit to ensure that the needed information is available before the consultation. Call several days prior to the appointment and check to see if her records have arrived. The consulting physician will share his or her opinion and send recommendations to the patient's physician, who can then take full advantage of the second opinion.

The most common benefit of a second opinion is having peace of mind in knowing that all of the needed information has been gathered to make an informed decision. An informed decision allows her to go through treatment knowing that this was the best treatment choice for her. Some women feel comfortable with their initial treatment options, feel their questions are answered sufficiently and feel no need for a second opinion. This is acceptable for them. Seeking a second opinion is an individual decision and one that needs to be made according to the patient's needs.

Remember...

Request written information from your healthcare team.

Obtain a copy of **Breast Cancer: Treatment Guidelines for Patients** *from the National Comprehensive Cancer Network.*

Take time to familiarize yourself with the terminology of breast cancer.

Second opinions may or may not be helpful in the decision-making process.

Accurate information is necessary to make treatment decisions. Only your physician and healthcare team can provide you with the specifics of the patient's diagnosis.

Communicate openly with the patient about the extent of your involvement during the decision-making process.

Support Partner

Two are better than one,
because they get a
good return for their work:

If one falls down,
his friend can help him up.

But pity the man
who falls and has
no one to help him up!

Also,
if two lie down together,
they will keep warm.
But how can one
keep warm alone?

Though one
may be overpowered,
two can defend themselves.

A cord of three strands
is not quickly broken.

Ecclesiastes 4: 9–12

Support Partner
Perspectives

"Anna had to decide what was the best surgical option for her. We discussed and researched the options at length, but she had to decide."

—Brian Cluxton, Support Partner

"My wife was not given the choice of surgical options because of her tumor size. In some ways not having to make this decision was easier on us."

—Al Barrineau, Support Partner

CHAPTER 11

Surgical Decisions

*U*sually, the first decision in the treatment of breast cancer is the type of surgical procedure to pursue. Breast surgery is the most effective method for treatment of breast cancer. Breast-conserving surgery, commonly referred to as lumpectomy or breast conservation, removes the lump and an area of surrounding tissue (margins). A mastectomy removes the entire breast.

Determining Factors for Type of Surgery

Surgery is the first line of defense against most breast cancers. The surgeon will discuss the best surgical options for the patient's diagnosis. Surgeons consider the following facts when determining which surgery, lumpectomy or mastectomy, is the most appropriate decision.

- **Type of Tumor**—The type was determined by a pathologist studying the biopsy specimen. There are approximately 15 cell types of breast cancer that vary in tumor growth rate (how aggressively the tumor may spread to other organs and its potential for occurring in the other breast).

- **Size of the Tumor**—Sizes are given in centimeters (cm) and millimeters (mm). (10 mm equal 1 cm; 1 cm equals ⅜ inch; 1 inch equals 2.5 cm)

- **Lymph Nodes**—Possible cancer involvement in lymph nodes.

- **Size of Breast**—Some breasts may be too small in comparison to the size of the lump to give good cosmetic appearance when the lump is removed.

- **Location in the Breast**—Tumors under the nipple sometimes will not give a suitable cosmetic look when the lump is removed. Two tumors in the same breast not located close to each other will not give good cosmetic results.

- **Mammogram**—Determines if the tumor may be multifocal (occurring within one quadrant in the breast) or multicentric (occurring in more than one quadrant in the breast). (Refer to graphic on page 126.) This is sometimes evidenced by microcalcifications (small calcium deposits) or mammographic abnormalities.

- **Involvement of Other Structures**—Skin, muscle, chest wall, bone or other organs.

- **Reconstruction**—Patient's desire for reconstruction now or later and the desired outcome for the reconstructive surgery (breast enlargement, reduction or matching present size).

- **Health**—General health and any treatment limitations due to present health.

- **Disease Control**—Which surgery will give the best chance for disease control.

- **Cosmetic Results**—Which surgery will give the best cosmetic results.

- **Range of Motion**—Which surgery will give the best functional results for her arm and shoulder.

- **Complications**—Which surgery is associated with the fewest short-term and long-term complications.

- **Personal Preference**—Her personal priorities regarding the surgery.

Each tumor must be evaluated in terms of its unique and specific features, as well as which surgery will be best for the patient. Some types of breast cancer may require neoadjuvant chemotherapy—chemotherapy treatments before surgery. This type of chemotherapy may be given to shrink a tumor to allow breast conservation (lumpectomy) with good cosmetic results.

Lymph Nodes

During the discussion about breast cancer surgery and treatment, the surgeon will talk about lymph node removal. Cancer that leaves the breast is often first found growing in the lymph nodes nearest the first node draining the tumor site. For this reason, lymph nodes are removed to determine whether the cancer has spread from the breast into the node area. Whether or not cancer is found in the patient's lymph nodes is one of the most important prognostic factors in breast cancer.

Evaluation of nodes for cancer cells is performed by a surgeon during breast surgery. Nodes may be evaluated by several methods: axillary sampling, complete axillary dissection or a procedure called sentinel lymph node mapping (if the tumor meets certain criteria). For identification purposes, nodes are divided into three levels in the underarm and chest area. (See graphic on page 127.) The number of nodes in each level varies from person to person.

Methods of Lymph Node Evaluation:

- **Axillary sampling** is a procedure in which selected nodes are taken from under the arm.

- **Axillary dissection** is a procedure in which all of the nodes under the arm are removed, usually from levels one and two.

- **Sentinel lymph node mapping** is a procedure that removes the first (sentinel) node(s) that drains the tumor for initial evaluation to see if additional nodes need to be removed.

Node Evaluation Results:

- **Negative nodes** mean that the lymph nodes did not have any evidence of cancer.

- **Positive nodes** indicate that cancer was found in the lymph nodes.

When the final pathology report is available, the surgeon will tell the patient how many nodes were removed during surgery and how many were found to have cancer cells present.

Sentinel Lymph Node Mapping

Sentinel lymph node mapping is a procedure that identifies the first (sentinel) node or nodes that receive lymphatic fluid from a cancerous tumor, thus identifying the lymphatic drainage pattern and the node(s) most likely to be cancerous. The sentinel nodes are like the gatekeepers to the rest of the lymph nodes.

Tumors may drain to different node chains according to the position of the tumor in the breast. The procedure identifies the lymphatic chain and the nodes most likely to indicate whether cancer has metastasized to the regional lymph node area. This identification gives the surgeon and pathologist a reliable guide for more accurate node evaluation without removing a large number of nodes. Not all patients are candidates for a sentinel lymph node procedure.

Sentinel Lymph Node Mapping Disqualifying Factors:

- Pregnancy
- Previous breast surgery in affected breast
- Known or suspicious positive lymph nodes
- More than one tumor in the breast
- History of breast radiation in affected breast
- Certain size tumors
- Ductal carcinoma in situ (surgeon's decision)

Sentinel Lymph Node Procedure

This procedure begins with an injection of a radioactive substance before going to surgery. Before surgery begins, the surgeon may also inject a blue dye around the tumor site or areola. The radioactive substance or dye is carried by the lymph fluid to the first node(s) (sentinel) that drains the tumor. During surgery, a hand-held gamma-detection probe first identifies where the radioactive material has concentrated, showing the area for the surgeon to make the incision. The blue dye helps the surgeon visually identify the node (there may be one or several) for removal. Some surgeons may only use the radioactive substance and gamma-detection probe, while others use only the blue dye. After surgery, the pathologist examines these nodes for cancerous cells.

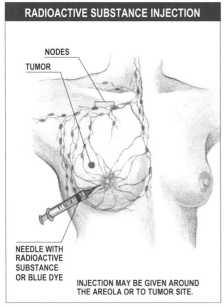

RADIOACTIVE SUBSTANCE INJECTION

NODES
TUMOR
NEEDLE WITH
RADIOACTIVE
SUBSTANCE
OR BLUE DYE
INJECTION MAY BE GIVEN AROUND
THE AREOLA OR TO TUMOR SITE.

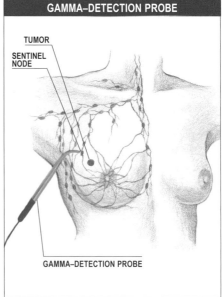

GAMMA–DETECTION PROBE

TUMOR
SENTINEL
NODE
GAMMA–DETECTION PROBE

If the sentinel node biopsy shows that there is no cancer, no additional nodes will be removed. If cancer is found in the biopsied node(s), additional node removal is necessary to determine how many nodes are positive. Additional node removal may be performed during the initial surgery, or at a later time. Some surgeons prefer to have the biopsy specimen evaluated during surgery, followed by additional node removal, if positive nodes are found. Others prefer to have the biopsy specimen evaluated later and, if the node(s) is positive, have additional nodes removed later. Ask the physician about the planned procedure for sentinel node evaluation.

Side Effects of Sentinel Lymph Node Biopsy:

- Pain during injection
- Bruising at the injection site
- Possible allergic reaction to the blue dye
- Bluish tint of the breast area or urine may occur if blue dye is used. The discoloration is temporary and is not harmful.

Sentinel node mapping improves the accuracy of selecting nodes to be removed surgically to check for the spread of the cancer. It may also prevent unnecessary removal of nodes not in the lymphatic drainage field of the tumor. Reducing the number of nodes removed can greatly decrease the potential for future lymphedema (a swelling from lymphatic fluid accumulation in the arm, which can cause discomfort and is a lifetime risk) and the likelihood of an infection in the arm if any type of injury should occur.

Treatment must be evaluated in terms of each tumor's unique and specific features and which surgery will be best for the patient. Some types of breast cancer may require chemotherapy treatments before surgery, called neoadjuvant chemotherapy. Discuss the above considerations with the surgeon and ask any questions that will help make the decision best suited to her needs.

Types of Surgery

Surgery for breast cancer includes several types of surgical procedures. Some types remove the breast (mastectomy), and others remove the tumor and varying degrees of the remaining breast tissue (lumpectomy). These common terms may describe various amounts of tissue removal. Ask the surgeon which of the exact procedures will be used. Following are the basic types of surgical procedures and descriptions of the tissues usually removed. After each description there are two drawings: one illustrates the amount of tissue removed, and the other illustrates how her body will appear after the surgery. Surgical incisions can vary among different surgeons.

Breast Conservation Surgery

Breast conservation surgery saves the majority of the breast tissue, including the nipple and the areola. However, there are some reasons that breast-conserving surgery may not be the best surgical option.

Disqualifying Factors for Breast Conservation Surgery:

- Pregnancy (if radiation therapy will be required before delivery; breast-conserving surgery is possible in the third trimester as long as radiation can be postponed until after delivery)

- More than one primary tumor in the breast

- Mammogram with evidence of suspicious scattered microcalcifications

- Location of the tumor in the breast where there may be poor cosmetic results (example: when the tumor is located under the nipple)

- Size of tumor (if the tumor is too large or the breast is too small in relation to the size of the tumor, then there will be poor cosmetic results)

- Prior radiation therapy to breast or chest area

- Collagen vascular disease (lupus, scleroderma, etc.)

- Severe chronic lung disease (because she may not be a candidate for radiation therapy)

- Very large, pendulous breast (may indicate that she may not be a good candidate for radiation therapy; she needs to have a radiation oncologist's evaluation)

- Evidence of remaining cancer in ducts surrounding the tumor after surgical removal (indicating there may be a high risk for recurrence)

- Inability of surgeon to obtain margins with no evidence of cancer after re-excision (second surgery)

- Possibly a positive carrier of a BRCA1 or BRCA2 mutated gene

- Restrictions on travel or transportation to clinic for daily radiation for six to seven weeks

Breast Conservation Procedures

Breast-conserving surgeries do not remove the breast and are commonly called lumpectomies. However, the term lumpectomy may be used inappropriately for other types of surgeries. These surgeries also conserve and do not remove the breast, but the cosmetic results and the amount of tissue removed can vary from procedure to procedure. These variations in the amount of tissue removed have different names which we will discuss below.

Lumpectomy

Lumpectomy removes only the tumor and a small margin of surrounding tissue. Lumpectomy preserves the basic appearance of the breast, including the nipple and areola. Lymph nodes may or may not be removed by a separate incision under the arm.

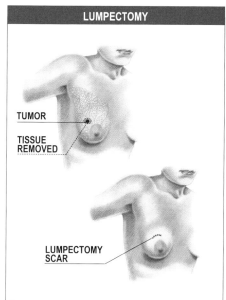

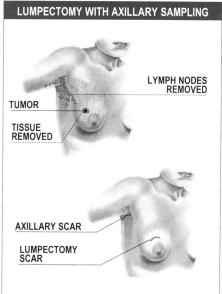

Wide Excision Breast-Conserving Surgeries

A surgery that removes more than just the tumor and a small amount of surrounding tissue may be called a partial mastectomy, quadrantectomy, segmental excision, wide excision or tylectomy. In these procedures, the tumor and an area of tissue around the tumor are removed. The overlying skin and a portion of the lining of the chest muscle under the tumor may also be removed.

These are all breast-conserving surgeries, but some may remove up to as much as 25 percent of the breast tissues. If it is necessary to remove a lot of tissue because of the characteristics of the patient's tumor, she may not be as pleased with the cosmetic results of the surgical procedure. Some of these surgeries may require some type of reconstruction, using an implant or her own body tissues, to restore her breast size. This is the reason she needs to inquire how much tissue will be removed. Ask her surgeon how much tissue will be removed.

Lymph Node Removal With Breast Conservation

Lymph nodes may or may not be removed from a separate incision, approximately two inches in length, under the arm. Lymph node removal during breast-conserving surgery also varies.

Potential Node Removal Types:

- No node removal
- Sentinel node biopsy
- Axillary sampling
- Axillary dissection

Ask the surgeon which type of lymph node evaluation procedure is recommended for her breast-conserving surgery.

Mastectomy Procedures

There are several types of mastectomies. Ask her surgeon which of the procedures will be performed and the extent of tissue and lymph node removal she will need to have. The different mastectomies are defined below:

1. Full or Complete Radical Mastectomy

A complete radical mastectomy removes the breast, nipple, areola, all three levels of lymph nodes, small chest muscle, the pectoralis minor, medial pectoral nerve and the lining over the chest wall muscles.

2. Modified Radical Mastectomy

A modified radical mastectomy removes the breast, nipple, areola, underarm lymph nodes and the lining over the chest wall muscles. The procedure may be referred to as a "total mastectomy with axillary dissection," which means that the entire breast and some or all of the level one and two lymph nodes are removed. Sentinel node mapping may also be used. This is the most common mastectomy.

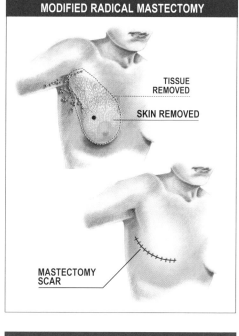

MODIFIED RADICAL MASTECTOMY

TISSUE REMOVED

SKIN REMOVED

MASTECTOMY SCAR

3. Total or Simple Mastectomy

This procedure removes the breast tissue, nipple, areola, and possibly some of the underarm lymph nodes that are closest to the breast or a sentinel node biopsy.

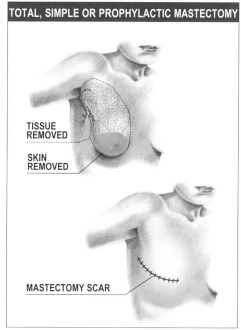

TOTAL, SIMPLE OR PROPHYLACTIC MASTECTOMY

TISSUE REMOVED

SKIN REMOVED

MASTECTOMY SCAR

73

4. Skin-Sparing Mastectomy

Skin-sparing mastectomy is a procedure used when performing a simple or total mastectomy. The method removes the breast tissues from a circular incision around the areola (dark colored circle). The nipple, areola, breast tissues, nodes located near the breast tissues and additional lymph nodes are removed according to the discretion of the surgeon. The procedure is often selected when reconstructive surgery is performed.

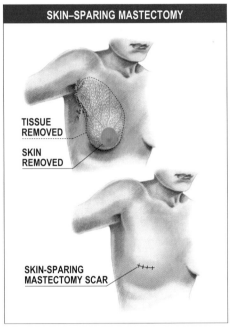

SKIN–SPARING MASTECTOMY

TISSUE REMOVED

SKIN REMOVED

SKIN-SPARING MASTECTOMY SCAR

The sparing of the skin allows reconstructive surgery to be performed with little need for a period of stretching the skin. Sensitivity of the skin over the reconstructed breast remains intact. The reconstructive incision is made using the normal curve of the breast. This incision is not visible because it is usually hidden under the fold of the breast and is concealed by the bra. The incision used to remove the breast is concealed by the reconstruction of a nipple and areola. This is the recommended surgery for women having mastectomy for intraductal disease and desiring reconstruction, or for a small peripheral tumor.

5. Prophylactic Mastectomy

A prophylactic mastectomy is a total or simple mastectomy performed before cancer has been found. This elective surgery is a decision made collaboratively between the patient, surgeon and oncologist. A second opinion may be required to ensure that this is a physically and psychologically sound decision.

Prophylactic Mastectomy Reasons:

- Desire for bilateral reconstruction with an increase or decrease in the reconstructed breast size

- Family history of breast cancer, including first degree relatives who died of the disease

- Identified positive carrier of BRCA1 or BRCA2 mutated genes
- Repeated breast biopsies for suspicious findings
- Mammograms that show findings which are increasingly difficult to interpret
- Diagnosis of a cancer type that has a high rate of occurrence in both breasts
- When the weight of a very large remaining breast (after mastectomy) creates imbalance, posture changes and back pain
- Overwhelming psychological fear of occurrence in remaining breast

Lumpectomy Versus Mastectomy

If the breast and tumor are within certain size limits, the surgeon may offer the option of a lumpectomy (breast conservation) versus a mastectomy. If the patient is in the category that allows her to choose between a lumpectomy and a mastectomy, the decision may be difficult. This needs to be a decision she makes in consultation with her physician after a careful review of the advantages and disadvantages of both. Remember, the option to choose is not available for some types of cancer.

It is imperative that she feels comfortable with the decision. Studies document that a lumpectomy, in an appropriate candidate, even if there is local recurrence, does not affect survival rate. However, it may be inconvenient if a second surgery becomes necessary. Ask the surgeon if there are any additional variables in the patient's surgical decision that may be added to this list.

Advantages of Lumpectomy:
- Saves a large portion of the breast, usually the nipple and areola
- Preserves body image
- Allows her to wear her own bras
- Rarely requires reconstruction or the wearing of a prosthesis, unless a wide excision lumpectomy was performed
- Recovery time from surgery is usually several weeks shorter than recovery from mastectomy
- Slightly shorter hospitalization time, or may be performed as outpatient surgery
- May be psychologically easier to accept, unless monitoring remaining breast tissue for recurrence is too frightening

Disadvantages of Lumpectomy:

- Risk of recurrence of cancer in remaining breast tissue (low risk)

- Several weeks, usually six to seven, of radiation therapy

- Changes in texture (lumpiness), color (suntanned appearance) and decreased sensation of feeling in the breast after radiation therapy

- Decrease in size of the remaining breast tissues after swelling decreases

- Monthly self-exam becomes more difficult because of increased nodularity

- Potential for chronic swelling or accumulation of fluid in the breast

- Possibility of future surgery if there is a recurrence

Advantages of Mastectomy:

- Removes approximately 95 percent of the breast gland, including the nipple and areola, thus reducing chance of local recurrence

- Reconstruction of breast is available using body tissue or synthetic implants

Disadvantages of Mastectomy:

- Body image changed because of the removal of a breast

- Need for prosthesis or reconstruction to restore body image

- Recovery time is usually several weeks longer than for lumpectomy patients

If the patient is having problems making a decision, she may wish to ask her physician if there is someone who will be willing to talk to her. The local American Cancer Society's Reach to Recovery program coordinator can provide the name of a volunteer who will be willing to share her lumpectomy/mastectomy experience.

If she is considering a lumpectomy, she may wish to have a consultation with a radiation oncologist to discuss radiation treatments. Often this consultation will give additional insight that may help her make a more informed decision.

*R*emember...

Surgical and reconstructive decisions need to be made by the patient, after she understands the advantages and disadvantages of each procedure.

Support Partner

A support partner
builds bridges of hope
and reassurance
when the one they love
is vulnerable,
exposed and
self-conscious.

A support partner
takes an interest in the patient,
but NOT
a controlling interest.

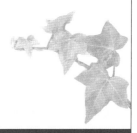

Judy Kneece

Support Partner
Perspectives

"The choice to have reconstructive surgery was not made easily. Helping my wife stand up for what she felt was best for her body took a lot of effort. I'm glad my wife sought my opinion, but the final decision had to be hers."

—Al Barrineau, Support Partner

"I don't recall having much of a 'say' in Anna's decision to do the TRAM reconstruction. Not because she didn't want me to have a say or my opinion didn't matter. I felt like it was her body and therefore her decision. I would support her, whatever she decided to do. We definitely talked about all of the different options, but ultimately she made the decision for the reconstruction she was most comfortable with."

—Brian Cluxton, Support Partner

CHAPTER 12

Reconstructive Surgery

Even though the patient may be losing a breast or a part of a breast to surgery, she has the option to have her body image restored through reconstructive surgery. Breast reconstruction has made a big difference, both physically and emotionally, for many women who have undergone surgery for breast cancer. Some have immediate reconstruction at the time of their initial breast surgery. They feel that reconstruction will help bring back their feminine silhouette and alleviate the necessity of wearing a prosthesis. Others wait until their treatments for breast cancer have been completed. Some women choose never to have reconstruction.

If the patient would like to have breast reconstruction, she should ask her surgeon for a referral to a reconstructive surgeon. A consultation with the reconstructive surgeon should take place before her cancer surgery, even if she plans to have delayed reconstruction.

A decision to have reconstruction requires a lot of research and discussion. Remember, part of her regaining control over cancer is understanding all of the options that are available and choosing those that best meet her needs. During this time of decision making, it is helpful if you remind her to ask herself, *"How would I like to look a year from now?"* This helps put her decisions into perspective.

Advantages of Breast Reconstruction:
- Restores feminine body image
- No prosthesis or special bras have to be purchased and worn
- Can wear any clothing, including swimsuits and low-cut attire
- Can go braless for short periods of time, if desired

- Does not have the daily reminder of breast surgery (in the form of a prosthesis)
- Psychologically beneficial in allowing most women to adjust better to the disease

Disadvantages of Breast Reconstruction:
- Physical recovery from surgery will require more time, and the patient will experience a greater degree of pain
- Increased potential for infection or surgical complications due to the more complex surgery

What May Disqualify a Patient?

Only a reconstructive surgeon can evaluate a patient's past and current physical condition to determine if she is a candidate for breast reconstruction and which surgery best suits her present health condition.

Potential Limiting Factors Are:
- Obesity (especially more than 25 – 35% over ideal body weight)
- History of radiation therapy to the chest wall
- Smoker or recent history of smoking
- Autoimmune disease (lupus, multiple sclerosis, insulin dependent diabetes mellitus, scleroderma, Hashimoto's thyroiditis, fibromyalgia)
- Current or previous history of chronic lung disease
- Psychiatric disorder
- Substance abuse
- Patient compliance (ability to understand procedures and options and the ability to tolerate pain from procedure)
- Abdominal scarring from previous surgery, including liposuction, if choosing a TRAM procedure (may prohibit use of abdominal muscle tissue in breast reconstruction)

The Good News

A woman is never too old for reconstructive surgery if she is in good health. Information about reconstruction and names of reconstructive surgeons can be obtained from the breast surgeon, Breast Health Navigator or nurse. Often, women fear that reconstruction may hide or prevent the detection of cancer recurrence in the breast area. There is no evidence of any kind that breast reconstruction, with her own body tissues or with an implant, causes cancer to grow or recur. There is little difficulty in detecting an early local recurrence after reconstruction. This should not be a concern in making a decision.

Reconstruction Reimbursement

In 1998, The Women's Health and Cancer Rights Act (WHCRA) was signed into law, providing coverage for the cost of reconstruction for women who elect to have a mastectomy. This law requires insurance providers to cover not only reconstruction of the surgical breast but also surgery, if needed, to the opposite breast to achieve symmetry (similar shape) between them. It also includes coverage for prostheses and any complications resulting from a mastectomy (including lymphedema, a swelling of the surgical arm). This law allows women to choose a mastectomy knowing that their reconstruction costs will be covered.

Immediate or Delayed Reconstruction

Reconstruction can be done immediately following cancer surgery, or it can be performed at a later time. There is no time limit after cancer surgery for reconstruction as an option to restore her physical image. The decision of when is the best time can be made by reviewing the advantages and disadvantages of immediate versus delayed reconstruction.

Advantages of Immediate Reconstruction:

- One surgery experience, requiring anesthesia (being put to sleep) only once
- Lower cost than two separate surgeries
- Reduced recovery time in comparison to two separate surgeries
- Body image does not suffer as great a change as has been associated with mastectomy alone
- Psychologically, there may be better adaptation

Disadvantages of Immediate Reconstruction:

- More physical discomfort and longer recovery time following surgery, when anxiety levels are at their highest
- Surgery using body tissues requires a much longer surgery and recovery time
- Surgery using implants requires only slightly longer surgery and recovery time
- Increased potential for infection or surgical complications which could delay treatments for cancer

Advantages of Delayed Reconstruction:

- Time to carefully study reconstruction methods and talk to patients who have experienced varying procedures

- Time to carefully select reconstructive surgeon and seek several consultations if needed

- Less psychological anxiety over cancer experience at time of reconstructive surgery

- No delay in treatments (chemotherapy or radiation) because of infection or complications from surgery

- Women who choose delayed reconstruction may be happier with their new breast than women who have immediate reconstruction because they have experienced the inconvenience of having to wear a prosthesis and the inability to go braless (thus their expectations were not as great)

Disadvantages of Delayed Reconstruction:

- Need for a second major surgery

- Higher cost because of second major surgery (anesthesia, surgery room, etc.)

- Cost of purchasing a prosthesis and special bras

- Inconvenience of having to wear a prosthesis until reconstructive surgery

- Temporarily unable to go braless or wear some low-cut clothing

- Procedure may fall into another deductible calendar year, requiring deductibles to be met for a second time

- Psychological distress from having to deal with an altered body image while waiting on reconstructive surgery

Types of Reconstruction

If the patient is considering reconstruction, an appointment for a consultation with a plastic surgeon to openly discuss her options will be helpful. After looking closely at her history, recommended surgical procedure (mastectomy or lumpectomy) and treatment recommendations (chemotherapy or radiation therapy), the plastic surgeon will take into account her desired reconstructive surgery outcome and make a recommendation.

There are many types of procedures available today which use implants or body tissue to reconstruct a breast. Implants may be filled with saline water, silicone or with combinations of both. Implants are placed under the chest muscle. Procedures called autologous reconstructions use body fat, with or without muscle, from the abdomen, back or buttocks to reconstruct a breast.

Surgical Procedure Decisions Depend On:
- Physical makeup (size of breast, degree of sagging)
- Physical health and history
- Preference for enlargement or reduction of the other breast during surgery

Breast Reconstruction Procedures

Breast Implants
Breast implants are the most common type of reconstructive breast surgery. The procedure may be done immediately after breast cancer surgery or later as outpatient or inpatient surgery. General anesthesia is usually used, and the surgery takes approximately one hour.

Indications for Implant Reconstruction:
- Women with small to medium-sized breasts, with little or no drooping (ptosis)
- Women with a small of amount of abdominal body fat
- Women desiring bilateral (both breasts) reconstruction
- Women not wanting additional scars
- Women who do not want longer, more complicated surgery
- Women in poorer general health or advanced age

Note: Women with large, drooping breasts who desire implant reconstruction usually require an additional surgical procedure on the opposite breast to match the size and contour of the breast implant.

Implant Procedures
There are two variations in implant procedures: (1) breast implant using an expander before final fixed-volume implant placement and (2) initial placement of a fixed-volume implant.

1. Breast Implants With Expander

Most women need to have their chest muscle and skin stretched before the final fixed-volume implant placement. An expander is inserted under the muscle and then gradually filled through a valve with a saline (salt water) solution every few weeks for 3 – 6 months. The surgeon injects about 50 cc of saline into the expander at each filling, causing slight discomfort for about 24 hours until the body adjusts to the new size. This gradual filling stretches the muscle and skin before the final implant placement. Additional surgery is required to remove the expander and position the fixed-volume implant.

A new combination expander and implant model allows the gradual expansion of the muscle and skin and does not have to be removed when the desired size is reached. The expander also serves as the permanent implant. Ask the reconstructive physician about this type of implant.

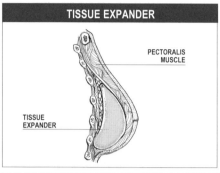

TISSUE EXPANDER

PECTORALIS MUSCLE

TISSUE EXPANDER

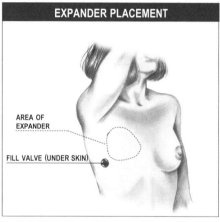

EXPANDER PLACEMENT

AREA OF EXPANDER

FILL VALVE (UNDER SKIN)

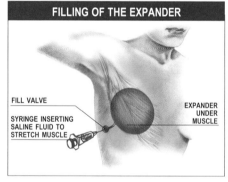

FILLING OF THE EXPANDER

FILL VALVE

SYRINGE INSERTING SALINE FLUID TO STRETCH MUSCLE

EXPANDER UNDER MUSCLE

2. Fixed Volume Implant

A soft shell filled with silicone gel or saline fluid or a combination of both is implanted under the skin and chest muscle. Surgery is either outpatient or inpatient and lasts approximately an hour. Local or general anesthesia may be used.

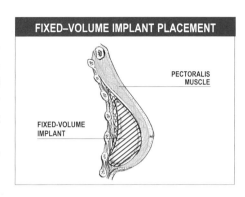

FIXED–VOLUME IMPLANT PLACEMENT

PECTORALIS MUSCLE

FIXED-VOLUME IMPLANT

Implant Advantages:

- Decreased surgical time for implant procedure
- Less pain after surgery than autologous body tissue reconstruction
- Decreased recovery time after surgery
- Decreased potential for surgical complications during and after surgery
- Less expensive surgery initially

Implant Disadvantages:

- An expander is usually needed to stretch out the muscles and skin before final implant placement. This requires multiple visits to the surgeon for injections of saline into the expander before final implant placement. During this time the surgical breast gradually matches the size of the other breast, unlike autologous (using body tissues) reconstruction, where the breast matches the other breast in size immediately after surgery.
- Expander fill-valve may malfunction, requiring replacement
- Final implant may leak or rupture, requiring replacement
- Difficult to match a large remaining breast with implants
- Radiation therapy after implant placement increases risk of complications
- Capsular contracture risk (tissues around implant harden and distort its shape)
- Contracture may cause pain, as well as visual change in shape
- Severe contracture may require removal of implant and placement of new implant
- Difficult to get reconstructed breast with implant to hang symmetrically on chest wall with opposite breast (implant cannot match natural droop of other breast)

- Implants will stay same size with weight gain or weight loss, unlike natural breasts

- Implants have a limited lifespan of between 10 to 15 years; they deteriorate and need replacement (potentially requiring future surgical procedures)

Saline Versus Silicone Implants

For the final implant, the patient will have to decide between a saline-filled or silicone-filled model.

Saline Implants:

- Saline implants are filled with sterile saline (salt) water that has the same concentration of salt as most body fluids, causing it to have no adverse impact on the body if it leaks or ruptures. The problem is that if it ruptures, it deflates within hours, causing the chest to appear flat.

- Ruptured implants have to be replaced in an additional surgical procedure.

- Saline implants are firmer when touched than silicone implants.

Silicone Implants

Silicone implants have been in use for over forty years. In the early 1990s, reports that ruptured implants might be causing autoimmune disorders caused the Food and Drug Administration (FDA) to investigate them, and for a period of time they were available only to breast cancer patients for reconstruction and not to women who simply wanted to increase the size of their breasts. The final conclusion by the FDA in 2006, after the Institute of Medicine researched the charge, was that there was no evidence of a link between currently available silicone implants and health disorders. Two brands of silicone implants were made available to anyone. Unlike the early implants, where the filling was the consistency of oil, the present implants' filling is very thick, like uncooked egg whites.

- Silicone implants are filled with a thick silicone filling that causes them to feel most like the human breast—softer to touch.

- Ruptured silicone implants can go undetected for years because the thick filling causes any leaks to be very slow—unlike saline leaks which are immediate. Surgical removal and replacement is recommended for leaking implants.

- The FDA recommends that women undergo magnetic resonance imaging (MRI) every few years to evaluate their silicone implants to detect any ruptures.

Comparison of Saline and Silicone Implants

	SALINE IMPLANTS	SILICONE IMPLANTS
Feels Natural	• Less able to mimic the feel of a natural breast	• Feels more like the normal breast
Size Variations	• Implant size can be increased or decreased after surgery during filling stage.	• Implant size cannot be changed after final implant placement. Implant is a fixed volume and is not filled by the surgeon.
Implant Rupture Potential	• Equal chance of rupture	• Equal chance of rupture
Ruptured Implant Symptoms	• Reconstructed breast deflates quickly as saline leaks into surrounding tissues and is absorbed. Patient is aware immediately that the implant has ruptured. • Replacement is required.	• Silicone gel leaks into the surrounding tissues but is not absorbed. Breast volume remains the same. Silicone implant ruptures may take longer to detect. • Replacement is required.
Replacement of Ruptured Implant	• Replacement is usually required at time of rupture, requiring an additional surgical procedure.	• Replacement is usually required at some point, requiring an additional surgical procedure.
Implant-Related Conditions	• Fibrosis or hardening of the tissues around the implant—called capsular contraction—may require surgery. • Infection • Pain • Nerve damage	• Fibrosis or hardening of the tissues around the implant—called capsular contraction—may require surgery. • Infection • Pain • Nerve damage

Autologous Reconstruction

Breast reconstruction using a woman's own body tissues (autologous) has many advantages, even with increased surgical complexity.

Advantages of Autologous Reconstruction:

- Avoids many complications relating to future surgical procedures for revision or replacement of implant

- Autologous tissues feel more like normal breast tissue, unless a woman is extremely thin

- Normal ptosis (drooping of breast) and inframammary crease (where the wire in an under-wire bra would be positioned) can be better matched by surgeon

- Surgeon can add additional skin flaps to avoid having to stretch skin if mastectomy scar is tight

- Post-surgical deformities or irregularities can be corrected with additional autologous tissues

- Donor sites (abdomen or hips) can have improvement in contour with reduction of body fat

- Lower cost over time because of fewer future complications and surgical revisions

- Volume and shape of autologous implants follow body weight changes

- Return of breast sensation is possible with certain types of reconstruction

- Breast feels warm when touched

- Provides solution for partial mastectomies or wide lumpectomies because of flexibility of tissues

- Preferred reconstruction if radiation therapy is to be part of cancer treatment

Disadvantages of Autologous Reconstruction:

- Requires sacrificing another body part to reconstruct your breast

- Additional time required for surgery

- Increased recovery time

- Increased pain after surgery

- Potential for tissue necrosis (cell death) of reconstructed breast from lack of blood supply to newly transplanted tissues, requiring removal and total loss of transplanted body part (Note: After surgery, the patient will be closely monitored for adequate blood supply to the newly transplanted tissues to detect any problems early and prevent loss of tissues.)

- Increased weakness in abdomen may limit physical activities and increase risk of hernia if abdominal muscles are used for reconstruction

Autologous Tissue Retrieval Sites And Reconstruction Types

- **Abdomen:**
  1. TRAM (Transverse Rectus Abdominis Myocutaneous muscle)
  2. DIEP (Deep Inferior Epigastric Perforator)

- **Back:**
  1. LD (Latissimus Dorsi)
  2. TAP (Thoracodorsal Artery Perforator)

- **Buttock:**
  1. Free superior or inferior gluteus
  2. S-GAP (Free-Superior Gluteal Artery Perforator)

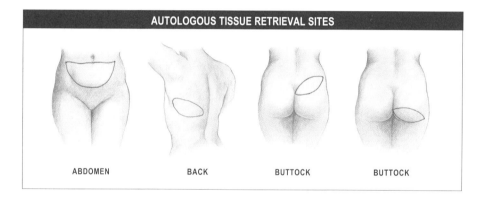

AUTOLOGOUS TISSUE RETRIEVAL SITES

ABDOMEN   BACK   BUTTOCK   BUTTOCK

Types of Reconstruction Flaps

If body tissues are used for reconstruction, the blood supply of the donor tissues moved to the breast area may be cut or left intact.

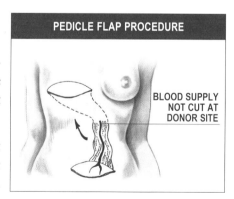

PEDICLE FLAP PROCEDURE

BLOOD SUPPLY NOT CUT AT DONOR SITE

- **Pedicle flap** is a procedure that moves the tissues, along with their own blood supply, to the breast area.

- **Free flap** procedure cuts the tissues of the selected area from their blood supply and reattaches them through microsurgery to blood vessels in the breast area. Free flaps are the most complex of all reconstructive procedures, requiring a surgeon with expertise in microsurgery.

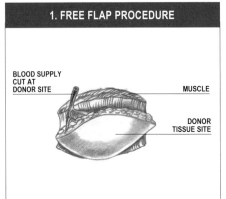

1. FREE FLAP PROCEDURE

BLOOD SUPPLY CUT AT DONOR SITE

MUSCLE

DONOR TISSUE SITE

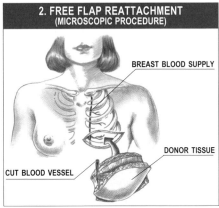

2. FREE FLAP REATTACHMENT
(MICROSCOPIC PROCEDURE)

BREAST BLOOD SUPPLY

DONOR TISSUE

CUT BLOOD VESSEL

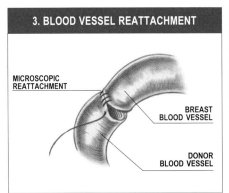

3. BLOOD VESSEL REATTACHMENT

MICROSCOPIC REATTACHMENT

BREAST BLOOD VESSEL

DONOR BLOOD VESSEL

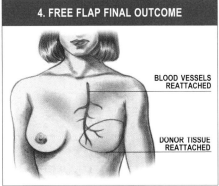

4. FREE FLAP FINAL OUTCOME

BLOOD VESSELS REATTACHED

DONOR TISSUE REATTACHED

Muscle-Sparing Reconstruction Flaps

Perforator flaps are recent refinements of conventional flaps where **none** of the underlying muscle is used. Perforator flaps can be taken from the abdomen (DIEP), back (TAP) or the buttocks (S-Gap). These procedures are relatively new. Ask your healthcare team if your reconstructive surgeons are skilled in these newer techniques.

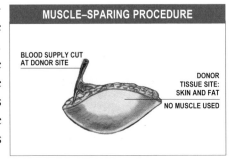

MUSCLE–SPARING PROCEDURE

BLOOD SUPPLY CUT AT DONOR SITE

DONOR TISSUE SITE: SKIN AND FAT

NO MUSCLE USED

Advantages of Perforator Flaps:
- Preserves muscle, which decreases the potential for future problems in donor site (weakness or restriction on activities)
- Preserving underlying muscle allows usual activities of daily living (sports, activities) as before surgery

Disadvantages of Perforator Flaps:
- Reconstructive surgeon experienced in new procedure is needed
- Prolonged operating time because of complexity of procedure

Three Major Types of Autologous Reconstruction

There are three major areas of tissue used for autologous reconstruction: abdomen, back or buttocks. Each of these sites may be left attached to the original blood supply (pedicle flap) or cut from blood supply (free flap). In addition, the muscle may or may not be used from each of the three sites.

Abdominal Tissue Procedures

1. TRAM Flap (Transverse Rectus Abdominis Myocutaneous muscle)

The transverse rectus abdominis myocutaneous muscle (major stomach muscle) is moved to the breast area with fat and skin and is attached to form a breast. This procedure is most commonly called a tummy tuck. This is the most common type of autologous flap used at present and is excellent for women with additional abdominal fat.

TRAM FLAP

PLACEMENT IN MASTECTOMY SCAR AREA

BLOOD SUPPLY NOT CUT

SKIN FLAP AND MUSCLE TUNNELED UP TO BREAST AREA

DONOR SITE: SKIN, FAT AND MUSCLE

Tram Flap Procedures:
- The transplanted tissue usually remains connected to its blood supply (called a pedicle flap), but occasionally tissues and muscle will be cut loose (free flap) and reconnected by microsurgery.
- Inpatient surgery with general anesthesia is required, lasting three to five hours and requiring several days of hospitalization.

- The procedure is moderately painful, causing difficulty in standing up straight for several days or weeks because of the cut muscle.
- Drains are usually removed after one week, but may be left in place for several weeks.
- A scar is left on the abdomen where the flap is removed.
- Disadvantages are an increased weakness of the abdominal muscle and wall, limiting strength and making some activities difficult, along with an increased potential for hernias.

2. DIEP (Deep Inferior Epigastric Perforator)

This procedure uses abdominal tissues without the abdominal muscle (rectus abdominis). The fat is harvested with local blood vessels (free flap, cut loose from local blood supply). Nerves can also be harvested along with the flap and used to restore sensation to the tissues when reattached in the breast area. Recovery time is reduced in this procedure compared to the TRAM flap because the muscle is not being moved, allowing earlier mobilization and return to normal activities.

Back Tissue Procedures

1. Latissimus Dorsi (back flap)

The back muscle (latissimus dorsi) and an eye-shaped wedge of skin are moved from the back and sewn in place on the breast area. The transplanted tissues are left attached to their original blood supply (pedicle flap).

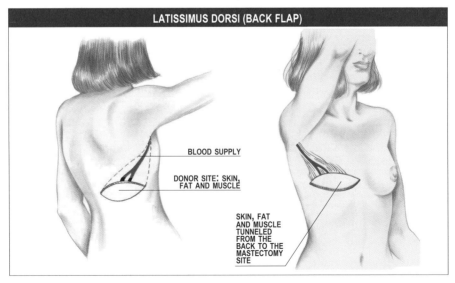

LATISSIMUS DORSI (BACK FLAP)

BLOOD SUPPLY

DONOR SITE: SKIN, FAT AND MUSCLE

SKIN, FAT AND MUSCLE TUNNELED FROM THE BACK TO THE MASTECTOMY SITE

This is an inpatient procedure with general anesthesia lasting two to four hours and requiring several days of hospitalization. The procedure is moderately painful, and a scar is left on the back. Drains may be left in place for several weeks. An implant, in addition to the patient's own tissue, may be required to match the opposite breast because of the size of the latissimus muscle moved. Some procedures can be performed endoscopically (using special instruments under the skin) without leaving a scar on the back. This procedure is excellent for small, non-drooping breasts or for partial, outer-quadrant reconstruction.

2. TAP (Thoracodorsal Artery Perforator)

This procedure is an alternative to the latissimus dorsi flap; it does not move the muscle, but uses the fat of the upper and lower areas around the muscle. Because some women do not have a lot of additional fat in this area, it may not be the preferred procedure.

Buttock Tissue Procedures
1. Inferior (lower) Gluteus (buttock) Flap

This procedure uses a patient's own tissue from fat and muscle in the buttocks. The tissue is detached (cut free) from its blood supply and reattached to the breast area blood supply using microsurgery. This is an inpatient procedure that includes general anesthesia. Surgery can range from three to eight hours, according to the degree of microscopic reattachment necessary. The scars on the buttocks are easily covered with underwear. Most women, except extremely thin ones, have tissue to spare.

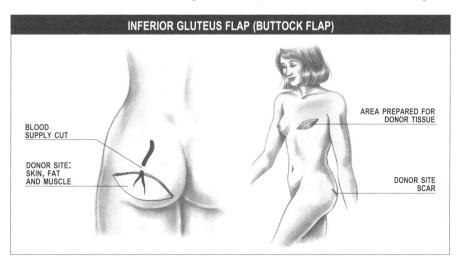

INFERIOR GLUTEUS FLAP (BUTTOCK FLAP)

BLOOD SUPPLY CUT

DONOR SITE: SKIN, FAT AND MUSCLE

AREA PREPARED FOR DONOR TISSUE

DONOR SITE SCAR

2. S-GAP (Free-Superior Gluteal Artery Perforator)

This is an upgrade of the gluteus flap; it requires no muscle to be harvested and only the fatty tissue and an artery for blood supply are moved to the breast and reattached using microsurgery. The tissue is removed from the upper portion of the buttocks (superior). This area has the potential to remove and transfer nerves to restore sensation to the new breast.

Nipple and Areola Reconstruction

1. The nipple and areola are usually reconstructed from existing skin and fat on the breast itself, or occasionally from tissues removed from other areas of the body, such as the groin.

2. The skin is molded to form the shape of the nipple.

3. The new nipple is sutured to the breast mound.

4. Areola reconstruction may be done by tattooing a dark pigmented color to match the other areola. Surgery is outpatient and pain is minimal.

NIPPLE AND AREOLA RECONSTRUCTION

1. SKIN FLAP

SURGEON CUTS SOME OF THE SKIN AND SOFT TISSUE ON THE BREAST MOUND TO FORM A NEW NIPPLE.

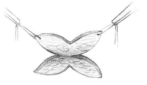

2. NIPPLE FORMED

SURGEON WRAPS TISSUES AROUND EACH OTHER TO FORM RECONSTRUCTED NIPPLE.

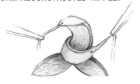

3. SUTURES

SURGEON SUTURES NEW NIPPLE IN PLACE.

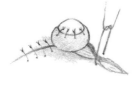

4. TATTOOING

AFTER THE NIPPLE HEALS, THE AREOLA IS ADDED BY TATTOOING TO MATCH THE OPPOSITE BREAST.

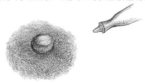

VARIOUS OTHER TECHNIQUES, INCLUDING SKIN GRAFTS FROM OTHER PARTS OF THE BODY, MAY BE USED. MOST OFTEN, THOUGH, SURGEONS USE A LOCAL SKIN FLAP. ASK YOUR SURGEON WHICH TECHNIQUE WILL BE USED.

The procedure is usually performed about six months after reconstruction when breast symmetry is satisfactory. Some women choose not to have their nipple and areola reconstructed after breast reconstructive surgery.

What to Expect After Autologous Reconstruction

Recovery Timeline:

- Someone will need to stay with the patient for several days when she returns home after surgery.
- Most patients can plan to return to work in 4 – 5 weeks, unless their job requires physical exertion.
- Swelling in the reconstructed breast and donor site where tissues were removed will persist for 1 – 2 months.
- Numbness in the reconstructed breast, donor site and sometimes the inner arm may occur for 6 – 12 months.
- Emotional letdown is normal for most women after breast reconstruction recovery and subsides when mobility returns.

Symptoms to Report to Physician:

- Temperature elevation above 100.5°
- Swelling that occurs quickly in breast or donor site
- Infection (redness, pus) in the area of incision or drain insertion site
- Change in color or temperature of reconstructed breast
- Pain that suddenly increases in the breast or donor site

Self-Care After Reconstruction:

- Sponge baths only until drains are removed. After drains are removed, the patient may shower. Water and mild soap are safe for the incision; however, do not scrub with a washcloth. No tub baths for two weeks.
- After a shower or bath, the surgical incisions should be allowed to dry before applying clothes or bandage.
- Change bandage as ordered by physician to keep area clean and dry.
- Prescribed antibiotics should be taken until all tablets are gone. Prescribed pain medication should be taken as needed, switching to extra strength Tylenol® or ibuprofen as soon as she is comfortable. The patient should not drive while on narcotic prescription pain medications.
- The patient should not drink alcohol while on prescription medication.
- No smoking or lifting of objects over 5 pounds for three weeks.
- No sleeping on the reconstructed breast or donor tissue site for three weeks; she should get out of bed on the side opposite her reconstruction.
- Daily walks are recommended.

Comparison of Breast Reconstruction Procedures

TYPE	ADVANTAGES	DISADVANTAGES	RECOMMENDED FOR	NOT RECOMMENDED FOR
Tissue Expander and Implant	• Short surgical time • Low initial cost	• Multiple fillings of expander with saline • 2nd surgery for implant • Capsular contracture • Leakage or rupture	• Medium size breast (400 – 800 cc) • Lumpectomy defect • Tight skin from radiation therapy	• Previous radiation therapy may limit size
Fixed-Volume Implant Only	• Short surgical time • One-step procedure • Lower initial cost	• Capsular contracture • Leakage or rupture	• Small breast (200 – 400 cc)	• Thin skin flaps • Radiation therapy
Latissimus Dorsi Flap (Pedical Flap) Muscle and Tissue	• Autologous tissues: skin, fat and muscle transfer • Small donor scar on back	• Muscle weakness • Potential seroma • Flap necrosis risk (1%)	• Small to medium size breast (400 – 600 cc) • Lumpectomy defect • Tight skin from radiation therapy	
TAP Thoracodorsal Artery Perforator (Free Flap) Tissues Only	• Autologous tissues: skin and fat only • No muscle removed • Small donor scar	• Potential seroma • Flap necrosis risk	• Small to medium sized breast (400 – 600 cc) • Lumpectomy defect • Tight skin from radiation therapy	• Extremely thin women
TRAM Flap Transverse Rectus Abdominis Myocutaneous (Pedicle Flap)	• Autologous tissues: skin, fat and muscle • Pedicle flap • Tummy tuck	• Scar on abdomen • Muscle weakness • Extended operative time • 6 – 12 wks. recovery • Abdominal wall hernia • Flap necrosis risk	• Mastectomy	• Previous abdominal surgery • Certain physical conditions • Cigarette smokers (some physicians)
DIEP Deep Interior Epigastric Perforator (Free Flap)	• Abdominal skin and fat only • Potential return of nerve sensations in area	• Additional scar on abdomen • Extended operative time from microscopic reattachment • Flap necrosis risk	• Mastectomy	• Previous abdominal surgery • Certain physical conditions • Cigarette smokers (some physicians) • Extremely thin women
Inferior Gluteus Flap (Free Flap)	• Autologous tissues: skin, fat, muscle and blood vessels removed from lower buttocks	• Scar at donor site • 6 – 12 weeks recovery • Extended surgical reattachment time • Flap necrosis risk	• Mastectomy	• Cigarette smokers (some physicians) • Extremely thin women
S-GAP Superior Gluteal Artery Perforator (Free Flap)	• Autologous tissues: skin and fat only • No muscle removed	• Scar at donor site • Shorter recovery • Extended surgical reattachment time • Flap necrosis risk	• Mastectomy	• Cigarette smokers (some physicians) • Extremely thin women

Complications and Risks of Reconstruction Procedures

COMPLICATION RISKS	MUSCLE-SPARING (FREE-TRAM OR DIEP)	NON MUSCLE-SPARING	IMPLANTS
Abdominal bulge or hernia	2 – 4%	5 – 10%	
Abdominal weakness	Virtually eliminated	30 – 60%	
Delayed healing	Less that 5%*	Less than 5%*	Less than 5%*
Premature removal related to rupture, capsular contracture or patient dissatisfaction			40% by 5 years
Free flap failure	2%	2%	
Replacement			10 – 15% at 10 yrs

*most common with previous radiation or smokers

To read explanations of DIEP and SGAP procedures, check timelines and see before and after photos, visit: **www.mauricenahabedian.com** and **www.diepflap.com**

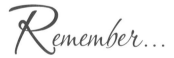*emember...*

A woman's body image can be restored using implants or her own body tissue after mastectomy.

If a woman is having a mastectomy, reconstruction is an option that she needs to investigate prior to her cancer surgery.

Reconstruction can be done immediately after cancer surgery or at any time in the future.

During decision making, remind her to ask, "How do I wish to look a year from now?"

Support Partner
Perspectives

"The hours in surgery were definitely the hardest time of the entire treatment period for me. I ended up walking around and around the hospital with my dad and my cell phone. I couldn't sit still, and it was good to have someone share my pain during this time."

—Brian Cluxton, Support Partner

"The early morning drive to the hospital was gloomy because of the cold and rain. We were both unusually quiet; each of us was locked in our own thoughts. This was the day we had dreaded, but now that it was here, we were ready to get it behind us. Just as we reached the hospital, the rain stopped and the skies cleared for a short time ... assurance the sun would shine again for us."

—Al Barrineau, Support Partner

"On the day of her surgery, I experienced partial relief from my fears for my mom. I knew surgery was necessary to rid her body of the cancer in her breast. Somehow, after surgery, I felt like the first part of our battle was behind us. Now, we had to move to the next battlefields: chemotherapy and radiation therapy. They still lay ahead of us."

—Krystle Brown-Shaw, Support Partner

Facing Surgery Together

The period between diagnosis and surgery is an anxious and exhausting time for a woman and her support partner. Before her surgery, the patient will be required to have a pre-admission assessment at the hospital or clinic. The physical assessment, which usually takes one to two hours, may include a chest X-ray, blood work, electrocardiogram (EKG) and instructions for surgery. Though not physically imposing, it is often emotionally distressing, and a time most women find a supporting person to be a great comfort. During the pre-operative workup, plan to have the following questions answered about surgery.

Surgery Questions:

- What is the last time the patient can eat or drink before surgery?
- What regular medications should she take the day of surgery?
- What time do we need to arrive?
- Where do we park the car on the day of surgery?
- Where does the patient report?
- Will her surgery require an overnight stay?
- Should we bring in personal items or wait and take them to the room, if admitted overnight?
- Where will I wait during surgery?
- How many people are allowed to wait in this area?
- Can I use my cell phone in the waiting area?
- How long is a patient usually in surgery?
- How long is a patient usually in recovery?
- Who will be relaying information to me concerning her condition?

- Will I be able to speak with the surgeon after surgery?

- What are the visiting hours in the hospital, if she is admitted overnight?

- Am I allowed to stay in the room overnight, if we so choose?

The Night Before Surgery

The night before surgery can be a very sad and stressful event for a woman. This is the last night with her body image intact. Some have to emotionally say goodbye to their breast as if it were an old friend. To ease her distress, plan to make this a special evening for both of you—a quiet, early dinner at her favorite restaurant or her favorite food at home. More important, however, is letting her know how special she is to you and that you are committed to be with her "no matter what comes." Give her space to work through this time in her own way with your silent support. While women will behave differently immediately prior to surgery, all appreciate a supportive, understanding person committed to them.

The Day of Surgery

You have both cried, fought the fears, looked for answers and confronted difficult decisions. On the day of surgery, both of you will probably be emotionally and physically drained. However, surgery often brings a sense of relief to the patient, through knowing that the cancer has been removed and that she may now go forward.

Allow enough time to arrive at the hospital without rushing. This is undoubtedly an emotional time for both the patient and you, the support partner. Most women may shed a few tears, are quietly withdrawn and visibly nervous about the surgery. Remember, what most women need is the presence of a support partner. There are no magical words or phrases to erase her fears, but your support will be what makes a difference.

Outpatient Surgery

Many women have outpatient surgery and return home after a stay in a recovery unit. In recovery, they are monitored until all of their vital signs (blood pressure, respirations, heart beats per minute, etc.) are in normal range, they are not vomiting and pain is controlled. The patient is then released to go home. Be sure you understand all discharge instructions before she leaves the hospital or clinic. Read the instructions given to you by her nurse. Ask for clarification, if needed. The patient may be awake and listening, but may not remember what is said because of the effects of the anesthesia. Ask for a name and telephone number that you may call if you have additional questions after you arrive home.

The Hospitalized Patient

If admitted to the hospital, the patient will be drowsy from anesthesia when she arrives in her room. Many women confess that they were not emotionally ready for many visitors the first day. If she feels this way, ask the nurse to place a "no visitors" sign on the door so that she can rest, and either shut off the telephone or answer the phone for her. Some women feel that this is a very personal time and would rather not have guests until they are feeling more in control of their emotions. Ask her what she would like for you to do to ensure she has adequate rest.

While the time spent in the hospital following surgery is usually very short, most women have said they appreciate the close presence of someone who cares about them. *"I didn't want to be left alone. Something inside of me felt as if I were a child again wanting someone to stay nearby,"* said one patient. This is an opportunity to offer the greatest of all support gifts—simply your presence. Your presence is definitely not medically necessary, but psychologically, it can be very valuable to the patient.

Getting the Facts

Following surgery, a new set of questions will surface. The best source for answers is the patient's physician and staff. Most physicians make their daily rounds to patients' rooms very early in the morning, before their office appointments begin. If possible, arrange to be in the patient's room at this time to ask the physician any questions. Make a list (samples on pages 102–103) so you do not forget what you need to ask. If the list of questions will require an extended amount of time to be adequately answered, schedule an appointment with the physician at the office. The nursing staff is also available to answer many of your questions. Physicians often have a nurse who is trained to answer basic questions.

Dressing Change

For patients staying overnight in the hospital, physicians often remove the surgical dressing and look at the incision the morning before the patient leaves the hospital. Ask if this is the policy of her physician. Those who have outpatient surgery will usually have their first dressing change during their first return visit to the physician.

Viewing the Scar for the First Time

I can tell you from experience, viewing the surgical scar during this dressing change is difficult for most patients. Seeing for the first time the missing breast because of mastectomy, or the surgically altered breast from breast conservation surgery, requires that she face the change in her new body image—a change no woman ever welcomes. This time, however, can be emotionally buffered when you, someone who cares about her, is there to share her experience. This is your role as a support partner—someone who stands alongside her, offering your presence as a source of comfort.

If you will be viewing the scar, the patient will be looking closely at your eyes to see your response at the first viewing of her new body image. To prepare for the viewing, it is helpful if she asks her nurse or physician to show her pictures of what the incision will look like prior to her surgery and viewing. These pictures or drawings will help both of you know how the incision area will look and remove some of the surprise by being prepared for what to expect.

Ask about the planned dressing change time so that you can plan to be there for her. During this first dressing change, the physician or nurse will explain what changes in the surgical area should be reported. If surgical dressing changes are recommended at home, instructions on how to change the dressing will be given. It is helpful if you listen carefully and ask for written instructions. Ask if surgical supplies can be sent home for these changes. If not, plan to purchases the supplies before needing them. Changing a surgical dressing on her own chest is difficult. This is something that you, as a support partner, can do that will be very helpful.

Preparing for Discharge

Before the patient is discharged, there are essential questions that she needs to ask to reduce anxiety about self-care at home.

Questions to Ask:
- How will pain be managed?
- What do we do if there is any nausea or vomiting?
- When, and what, can the patient eat?
- When can regular medications be resumed?

- If she has bulb drain(s) inserted during surgery to remove fluid accumulation at the surgical site, when and how should they be emptied? (Ask for a demonstration, if not previously given.)

- Should the amount of drainage be recorded? (Be sure you understand how to measure and record the amount.)

- To what extent can the surgical arm be used?

- Does the surgical arm need to be propped up on a pillow while she is lying down?

- Should the surgical dressing be changed before we return to the physician? (If yes, ask for detailed instructions and for supplies to take home.)

- When can a bath be taken? What type of bath?

- When can she shampoo her hair?

- What symptoms need a physician's immediate attention? (Bleeding, increased pain, clogged drains, fever, etc.)

- When does an appointment need to be scheduled with the physician? (Do we call for an appointment, or has one already been made?)

- When does she get the final pathology report?

For support partners involved in an intimate sexual relationship, refer to Chapter 18, "Sexuality After Breast Cancer."

*R*emember...

Accompanying the patient to her pre-admission workup is psychologically comforting.

The night before surgery is a highly emotional time for most women. Careful, sensitive planning can make it easier for both of you.

Most women need extra support prior to and immediately following surgery.

Ask for clear discharge instructions.

Support Partner
Perspectives

"Talking about hard things, even her own breast cancer, was easy for Mom. She was open and talked about it; it was no big deal for her to tell me what she was thinking and feeling. This made it easier for me. It opened the doors for me to talk, knowing that we could discuss things openly and not hide our thoughts and feelings from each other. We did not play emotional 'hide and seek' with each other."

—Krystle Brown-Shaw, Support Partner

"After surgery she needed to talk and talk. I had never known her to talk so much. She drew comfort from my response, even when it was only a nod of agreement. Listening to her fears, her hopes, and sharing her tears was what she wanted most. At times, I didn't want to hear what she was saying. I wanted to hide in the newspaper or television, but I knew she needed me. I'm glad I took the time to listen."

—Al Barrineau, Support Partner

"I really had to work hard to listen and not try to 'fix' it."

—Brian Cluxton, Support Partner

CHAPTER 14

Resuming Communications...
What Do I Say?

Some support partners find it painful to talk about the cancer or the surgical experience. One patient lamented about her husband, *"Losing my breast was not nearly as hard as losing my mate emotionally. ... He wouldn't talk about it after surgery. He stayed away from home except when he was eating or sleeping. ... When I tried to talk about my cancer experience, he just looked at me and would not say anything."*

David Spiegel, M.D., conducted a study of families with cancer to determine what families can do that best helps ailing loved ones cope with their illness. He concluded:

We found that certain types of family interaction at home predicted how well the sick member of the family felt over time. The more family members supported one another, talked openly about problems and reduced conflict, the happier the sick members were. In particular, expressiveness, a measure of shared and open problem solving, seemed to be a reliable predictor of how both sick and well family members would cope with a variety of illnesses. The lesson is that it pays to solve problems together rather than struggle with them separately. Our tendency is to hide what worries us from ourselves and from those close to us. This (hiding worries) creates isolation, impairs problem solving and seems to make sick people sadder and more anxious. While it may be true that 'misery loves company,' it seems that company dispels misery.

Talking About Cancer Can Be Hard

Communicating after breast surgery can be difficult for both the patient and the support partner. Many find it hard to express their thoughts, fearful that they may hurt the other's feelings or that they may "lose it" emotionally. Barriers are often erected to prevent communication from occurring. The most common barrier is emotional withdrawal—silence.

Silence: An Emotional Retreat

Emotional seclusion becomes a safe retreat. The workplace or a hobby often becomes a safe place to hide. Being absorbed in work often becomes the antidote for emotional pain. To the patient, this withdrawal or silence may be perceived as rejection or withdrawal of your love. This may cause her to become angry—expressed or internalized—and can eventually lead to depression. This emotional trauma can usually be avoided through early, honest communication. You must talk! You must listen! While painful at first, it is necessary for an emotional recovery from breast cancer. Communicate your feelings to each other—anger, fear and sorrow— whatever they may be. Don't push or force the issue, but realize that **not** talking about cancer may be as dangerous to a relationship as cancer is to the physical body.

Understanding Her Real Needs

Understand that she needs to feel free to express her thoughts without judgment from you. Patients know there are no perfect answers; they just need to talk. Many times a woman needs to say the same thing over and over, so the best advice is just to listen. Do not be afraid of hearing about her fears and feelings or seeing her tears. Remember, tears are a sign that she is in touch with reality and is successfully grieving her loss. Your tears are not a sign of weakness and will not weaken your relationship. One woman shared, *"For the first time in my life, I saw the tears in his eyes as we talked about my surgery, and I knew without a doubt that he felt what I was feeling. Somehow, from that point on, I knew we were going to make it together."* Tears have a language of their own and often say what we could never verbalize. They prove to the other person that we are emotionally in touch with their pain and share their sorrow.

Soliciting Her Needs

Communicating is difficult for some. They feel as if they don't know what to say. Spoken under stress, words often become even more powerful and may even be misinterpreted. Being stressed over the future is a normal part of a cancer diagnosis. Needing to share concerns and worries is a vital part of coming to terms with natural fears and helps her sort out options. Helping her feel comfortable talking with you requires that you listen attentively and know how to ask questions that give her permission to continue to share her real fears and feelings.

Your goal is to solicit information from her. You can do this by asking open-ended question such as: *"Tell me how you feel about _____."* *"Share your thoughts about this decision with me."* These open-ended questions allow the doors of communication to be opened. Some women need this verbal invitation to share their thoughts and feelings. They are not going to talk about their cancer until they are given permission and they know that they have a safe place to share without someone being judgmental or critical of their innermost thoughts and fears.

Open-Ended Statements and Questions to Encourage and Promote Good Communication:

- Tell me about what happened to you.
- Go on … tell me more.
- Give me an example of what you mean when you say _____ .
- Describe that further for me.
- Describe how you felt when that happened.
- Please explain that to me; I want to better understand how you feel.
- Explain the details in the order that you remember them.
- Help me understand what you mean when you say that.
- How important was that to you?
- What do you think the reason was for that to occur?
- What do you see as the problem?
- What do you mean when you say that?
- If I heard you correctly, you said (repeat statement).
- Is this what you were saying/feeling?
- What would you do if this situation occurs again?
- What would you want to happen if this situation occurs again?

Listed below are barriers to communication, along with helpful and non-helpful responses. Read them carefully to see if there are any areas that may improve your communication skills with your partner.

Therapeutic Communication Guidelines

BARRIERS	NOT HELPFUL	HELPFUL
Giving Advice	Why don't you ___?	Have you considered ___ at this time?
	If I were you, I would ___.	What do you think would work best for you?
	You need to ___.	A good option to think about is ___. Some women find ___ helpful.
False Reassurance	Don't you worry!	What worries you most about this situation?
	Everyone feels like that.	Tell me what you are feeling.
	Things look worse before they get better.	This must be a very hard time for you. How are you handling this emotionally?
	This will be a piece of cake.	You seem to have all of the qualities it takes to do well during treatment.
Changing the Subject	Let's talk about that later.	That sounds important. Tell me more.
Judgmental Attitude	You are wrong about that.	You understand this differently than I do. How do you see the situation?
	Don't think like that!	Tell me what you are thinking now.
	That's not a good decision when you have cancer.	I may not agree with your decision, but I understand where you may be coming from.
Direction Giving	This is the way you should do this.	Which of these ways do you think would work best for you?
	You need to/must follow the instructions.	Let's look at different options you have. How would you handle the situation?

BARRIERS	NOT HELPFUL	HELPFUL
Emotionally Charged Words	Your doctor/nurse/mother/child makes you very angry.	How do you feel about what he/she did?
	I'd tell them to mind their own business if they ask.	Do you mind people being inquisitive about your illness?
	Your doctors should not say that to you!	What do you think about what he/she said to you?
Challenging	You can't do that yet!	It sounds like you think you may be well enough to ___ now. Do you think that is wise?
Trite, Stereotyped Expressions	You look chipper!	Gee, you're smiling a lot today, does that mean you're feeling better?
	Things always look better in the morning.	How hard is it for you to keep going during chemotherapy?
	No pain, no gain!	Dealing with pain is tough; how are you handling all of this?
	Bald is beautiful, you know!	Hair loss is the hardest side effect for many people during treatment; how are you feeling about it?
	It is better to lose a breast than to lose your life.	The loss of a breast must be very hard to deal with. How are you feeling about your surgery?
	Breasts aren't necessary for good sex.	Some women have trouble feeling sexy after breast surgery. How are you feeling?
Value Statements	You just need to have faith.	I know this is hard. This is testing my faith, too.
	Relax. God is in control.	Sometimes it's hard to feel God's presence.
	You just need to pray and let this fear go.	Can we pray about this together?

The Magical Communication Skill

At times when you don't feel adept at using words to convey your concern, there is another powerful, almost magical, option. It is your non-verbal body communication. You can convey much by the way you physically respond to the patient during this time. In fact, experts say that body language is a stronger indicator of how someone feels than the words they say. Use this powerful tool to enhance your communication. Instead of words, use your body language to let her know how you feel.

Non-Verbal Communication Support Options:
- Hold her hand.
- Make direct eye contact.
- Place your hand on her shoulder.
- Pat her on the back.
- Sit or lie close to her.
- Lean forward toward her when she is speaking.
- Wink at her, when appropriate, if you catch her eye in public.
- Seek out her presence in a crowd.

There are numerous other non-verbal ways you can convey your support without saying a word. Remember, a very large part of your communication to her during this stressful time is from your body language. It can relay your concern, support and love when you can't find the right words to say.

Interpreting Her Body Language

The other part of communication enhancement is learning to read her body language.

Carefully Observe Her Body Language for Signs of Personal Need:
- Look at her eyes for signs of distress
- Frowns for signs of disapproval
- Squinting of eyes for a desire to better understand
- Tears for signs of feelings of loss, helplessness or aloneness
- Questioning stares as a need for additional information
- Slumped posture as a sign of discouragement
- Closing of eyes as a sign of discouragement or emotional withdrawal

- Failure to make eye contact, as a sign of desire to avoid a person
- Repetitive movement of arms and legs or tapping of fingers as a sign of high anxiety

When you observe her body language, you can then clarify her needs with statement such as, *"I feel that you may be tired (upset, concerned or confused). Is this an accurate observation?"* Observing her body language and verbalizing these observations conveys absolute recognition of her needs and allows her to verify or communicate previously unspoken concerns.

Clear Communications: A Tool for Recovery

Effective communication and support from a support partner is one of the best tools for recovery. In fact, women in our focus groups rated their need for support as high as their need for medical treatment during breast cancer. Direct, sensitive communication between partners in a caring non-judgmental manner enables a healthy acceptance and problem-solving approach, facilitating the emotional recovery from breast cancer.

During a crisis, communication skills become extremely important. The patient faces a multitude of decisions, changes and losses at this time. She is forced into stressful situations. Your ability to allow her to express her feelings in an atmosphere of understanding, rather than judgment, can powerfully influence her ability to cope. Effective communication skills alleviate additional stress as well as help to resolve situations as they arise. Remember that communication is not just talking, but also the art of listening well.

When She Talks:

- Look directly into her eyes.
- Turn off the television, put down the paper and avoid checking the phone or texting.
- Don't constantly look around to see what others are doing.
- When she has stated what she needed to say, clarify what she meant if you are uncertain.
- Ask open-ended questions to encourage her to tell you more.
- Respond with statements that reflect your respect for her opinions, fears or questions.

If Something She Says Upsets You:

- Stop and take a deep breath.

- Think about "why" you are upset about what she said.

- Do you feel compelled to stop her hurt and make everything all right?

- Do you feel a need to "win" this point of difference?

- Do you feel that you need to set her straight on the facts?

- Do you feel there would not be a problem if she just did what you told her to do?

- Are you afraid to show any sign of weakness?

- Do you feel you just don't want to hear all of this again?

- Determine why her words created stress in you, and then carefully choose how you respond.

Choosing to be an effective support partner is a choice you constantly make. Often this requires practicing new skills of communication. The patient's point of view is expressed in *I Need A Heart to Talk To* on page 113.

*R*emember...

Communication is even more essential after breast cancer.

Women listen intently to what you say (and don't say) and observe your body language. Be careful not to send mixed messages.

Listening is an important part of communication. Let her talk. Talking can be therapeutic.

I Need a Heart To Talk To

I need to talk—and all I ask is that you listen to me.

Somehow, when my heart pours forth its thoughts,
fears and worries, they lose some of their power over me.

When you stop me with,
"You shouldn't feel that way," or *"Don't say that,"* advice,
you push the power of their terror back deep into my heart.

Where once again, in the dark of night, the power of their
terror engulfs my spirit with fear and confusion.

You say you want to help.
I just need a heart to listen to me when I need to talk.

I don't need "head advice."
I just need a heart to intimately share the moment.

I need a heart that feels, for a few seconds, what I feel.

I need a heart that shares my sorrows with compassion.

I need a heart that recognizes my fears as
my own struggle to face the unknown.

I need a heart of trust, so that when I pull out the terror
inside of me, I feel that it will be allowed to dissipate
in the clean air of another caring heart.

When all is said and done, what I am asking for is
your heart of understanding when I talk.

I don't need any more "head advice."

Somehow, heart listening is a
more powerful medicine to my spirit.

Judy Kneece

Support Partner
Perspectives

"*Surgery produced a lot of stress and anxiety. Then came another stressor, the final pathology report. This was the report that contained the secrets of what was in her body and would direct her future treatment. Yet, it was very difficult for me as a lay-person to understand. The answer was in having a doctor explain the report in terms we could understand. So, don't let it confuse you: ask a physician to explain it to you. ... In the beginning, I thought my wife would die. I thought breast cancer was a death sentence. When the physician explained the particulars of her pathology report, it gave us a renewed hope that our dreams for the future could still be realities. We were told the factors that were significant for her prognosis. Several things in the pathology report helped us know that her cancer was part of a large disease, but was also uniquely hers. We could draw strength from others, but we could not make comparisons.*"

—Al Barrineau, Support Partner

"*The final pathology report showed that Mom would need to have chemotherapy to treat her cancer. This report confirmed what the doctors had predicted before her surgery was indeed accurate. Chemotherapy would be the next step. The pathology report was the roadmap for the physicians to be assured the right drug was being given to her. Thank goodness doctors have a guide for making these decisions.*"

—Krystle Brown-Shaw, Support Partner

114

CHAPTER 15

Understanding the Pathology Report

T he preliminary pathology report received after the patient's biopsy contained a lot of information about her cancer. A final pathology report will be prepared after the final cancer surgery that will give additional information about her cancer and the status of cancer in the lymph nodes. Her treatment plan is based on both the preliminary and the final pathology reports. From this series of reports, her physicians will determine which course of treatment is best suited for her individual case. The most common treatments are chemotherapy, radiation therapy and hormonal therapy. Treatment may consist of one or more types of treatment. For some women, no further treatment may be needed after surgery beyond close observation by the physician. Because of the wide variety of treatment plans, her physician will provide specific information regarding her planned treatment.

The Pathology Report

Because treatment decisions will be based on the pathology reports on the tumor, it may be helpful to understand how the reports are used in determining treatment options. However, it is not essential to understand all of the following information. Some people feel that this is more information than they want to know. Feel free to skip this section. It is included in case you need to clarify questions about the pathology report.

After the tumor was removed from the patient's breast, it was sent to a pathology laboratory where it was carefully processed. There, a pathologist (a physician who specializes in diagnosing diseases from tissue samples) analyzed the tissues by careful, naked-eye dissection as well as under a microscope and issued a pathology report to her physician. This report contains the unique characteristics of her individual tumor. This report will help her physicians determine if she needs additional treatment. If additional treatment is needed, the pathology report will be used as a guide for all of her physicians to develop a treatment plan for her cancer.

The slides and tissue blocks prepared by the pathologist to study the tumor may remain available for additional consults and future studies if research unfolds new tissue diagnostic tests.

Characteristics of Cancer Cells

- **Normal Cells**—Normal ducts and lobules are lined with one or more layers of cells in an orderly pattern.

- **In Situ Cancer**—It is called "in situ cancer" when these normal cells become abnormal and cancer develops and grows. In situ cancer does not break through the wall but remains in the duct or lobule where it began. This type has a good prognosis.

- **Invasive (Infiltrating) Cancer**—Cancer that has broken through the wall of the duct or lobule and has begun to grow into surrounding tissues in the breast is considered invasive or infiltrating cancer. "Microinvasive" means that just a small amount of cells have grown through the duct or lobular walls.

Types of Breast Cancer

The most common types of breast cancer are listed below. There are also various other rare types of breast cancer and combinations of the following types.

- Infiltrating (invasive) ductal (approximately 52% of patients)
- In situ ductal (intraductal) (approximately 21%)
- Invasive lobular (approximately 5%)
- In situ lobular (intralobular) (approximately 2%)
- Medullary (approximately 6%)
- Mucinous or Colloid (approximately 3%)
- Paget's disease with intraductal (approximately 1%)
- Paget's disease with invasive ductal (approximately 1%)

Remaining Cancers Occurring in 1% or Less:

- Tubular
- Adenocystic
- Cribiform
- Inflammatory
- Papillary
- Carcinosarcoma
- Micropapillary
- Squamous
- Apocrine
- Sarcoma

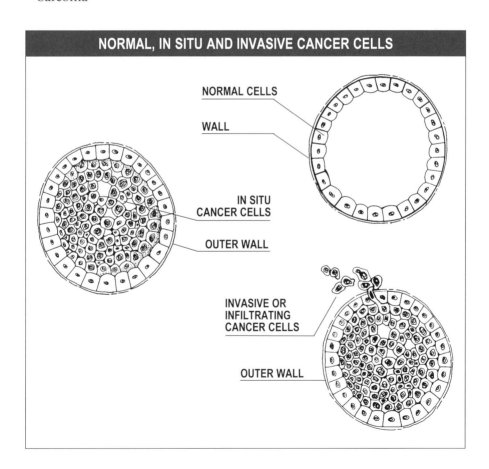

NORMAL, IN SITU AND INVASIVE CANCER CELLS

Tumor Size

Tumor size is the measured size of the tumor. Results are reported in millimeters (mm) or centimeters (cm).

- 10 mm equals 1 cm
- 1 cm equals ⅜ inch
- 1 inch equals 2.5 cm

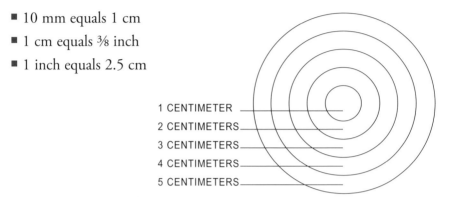

1 CENTIMETER
2 CENTIMETERS
3 CENTIMETERS
4 CENTIMETERS
5 CENTIMETERS

Tumor Shape

The report may also state the shape of a solid tumor as being round, spherical or having irregular contours such as stellate or spiculated.

Margins

Margins are the area cut by the surgeon's knife surrounding the tumor.

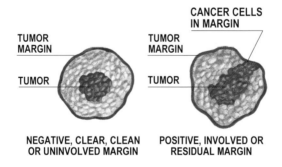

CANCER CELLS IN MARGIN

TUMOR MARGIN

TUMOR

TUMOR MARGIN

TUMOR

NEGATIVE, CLEAR, CLEAN OR UNINVOLVED MARGIN

POSITIVE, INVOLVED OR RESIDUAL MARGIN

Terms to Describe Pathology Margins:

- **Negative, clear, clean or uninvolved:** means there was no evidence of cancer cells in the margins.

- **Positive, involved or residual cancer:** means that cancer was found in the margins.

- **Indeterminate:** means the pathologist could not determine and make a definite statement about the margins.

Node Status

If surgery included lymph node removal using sentinel node or axillary dissection, the report will state how many nodes were removed, a description of the area from which the nodes came and how many nodes tested positive for cancer cells.

- **Lymph node negative:** means no cancer was found in the lymph nodes.

- **Lymph node positive:** means that cancer was present in the lymph nodes.

Nuclear Grade

Nuclear grade evaluates the size and shape of the nucleus in tumor cells and the percentage of tumor cells that are in the process of dividing or growing. Cancers with a low nuclear grade (Grade 1) grow and spread less quickly than cancers with a high nuclear grade (Grade 3).

Grading of Tumor

The general grading of cells is a microscopic examination of the cells that shows the degree of change from normal. The pathologist observes how much the cells resemble the original cells.

Tumor Cells Are Graded or Classified As:

- **Undifferentiated cells**—These cells have an abnormal appearance and have changed greatly from the cell from which they originally developed. Usually most aggressive. High grade (Grade 4).

- **Poorly differentiated cells**—These cells have lost most of the characteristics of the cell from which they came. Usually aggressive. High grade (Grade 3).

- **Moderately differentiated cells**—These cells have changed but still resemble the parent cell. This term is used to describe cells between the well differentiated and poorly differentiated stages. Moderately aggressive. Intermediate grade (Grade 2).

- **Well differentiated cells**—These cells are very similar in appearance to the cell from which they evolved. Usually least aggressive. Low grade (Grade 1).

USC/Van Nuys Prognostic Pathologic Classification — Ductal Carcinoma in Situ

Treatment for ductal in situ carcinoma (DCIS) is undergoing change. Some physicians use the USC/Van Nuys Prognostic Pathologic Classification to determine if a patient could be a candidate for breast conservation rather than mastectomy according to various pathological studies performed on the tumor. In this pathologic evaluation, four categories are observed and a score is given to each category. The total score is used to determine who may qualify for various treatments. Ask if her physicians use this method of evaluation for DCIS. Many experts use other means of evaluation.

1. Nuclear Grade	Grade Value	
Non-high grade without necrosis	1 point	Evaluates size and shape of nucleus of cells
Non-high grade with necrosis	2 points	
High grade with necrosis	3 points	

2. Tumor Size	Grade Value	
1.5 cm and under (<14 mm)	1 point	Evaluates size of the area where DCIS is found
1.6 cm to 4.0 cm (15 – 40 mm)	2 points	
4.1 cm or greater (>40 mm)	3 points	

3. Tumor Margins	Grade Value	
1.0 cm or greater (>10 mm)	1 point	Evaluates distance from DCIS to margins of surgical specimen
0.1 – 0.9 cm (1 – 9 mm)	2 points	
0.1 cm or under (<1 mm)	3 points	

4. Age at Diagnosis	Age Value	
Over 60	1 point	Factors in age at diagnosis
40 – 60	2 points	
Under 40	3 points	

Final Cumulative Total	
4 – 6 points = no difference in survival-free local recurrence after lumpectomy with/without radiation therapy	Total of the scores in the above four areas determines final grade
7 – 9 points = significant decrease in local recurrence with radiation therapy	
10 –12 points = high rate of local recurrence; mastectomy recommended	

The Scarff/Bloom/Richardson/Elston Grading Scales

Some pathologists use the Scarff/Bloom/Richardson scale or a slight modification called the "Elston Grade" for grading invasive tumors. These grading systems give a number from 1 to 3 according to aggressiveness of three different characteristics of the tumor: (1) tubular formation, (2) nuclear size/shape and (3) cell division (or proliferation) rate.

The numbers from each characteristic are then totaled to determine the aggressiveness of a tumor. The higher the number, the more aggressive the characteristics of the tumor.

1. Tubular Formation	Grade Value	Evaluates cell arrangement for characteristics of looking like a small tube
Majority (>75%)	1 point	
Moderate degree (10 – 74%)	2 points	
Little or none (0 – 9%)	3 points	

2. Nuclear Shape/Size	Grade Value	Evaluates size and shape variation of cells and nucleus of cells
Uniform, small nuclear shapes	1 point	
Moderate increase in size and varying shapes	2 points	
Marked abnormalities (often large nucleus)	3 points	

3. Cell Division Rate	Grade Value	Determines how many cells are visible in the dividing stage in an area of the tumor
Low (0 – 5)	1 point	
Moderate degree (6 – 10)	2 points	
High (>11)	3 points	
*Cell Division Rate (Elston Grading Scale Modification) Grade Value		*These numbers vary according to the Elston Grading Scale.
Low (0 – 9)	1 point	
Moderate degree (10 – 19)	2 points	
High (>20)	3 points	

Final Cumulative Total	Points	Total of the scores in the above three areas of evaluation determines final grade
Grade 1 – well differentiated	3 – 5 points	
Grade 2 – moderately differentiated	6 – 7 points	
Grade 3 – poorly differentiated	8 – 9 points	

121

Prognostic Tests

Various tests may be performed on the tumor by the pathologist to look at specific characteristics of the tumor cells.

- **Flow Cytometry**—A test that looks at the genetic material found in the DNA of a cell. Normal DNA of a cell has two sets of chromosomes. **Diploid** means having two sets of chromosomes, which is normal. **Aneuploid** refers to the characteristic of having either fewer or more than two sets of chromosomes.

- **Cell Proliferation Rate**—Flow cytometry can also identify the number of cells dividing, called the S-phase fraction. This information allows a physician to know approximately how rapidly the cancer was growing (mitotic rate) at the time of surgery. A high S-phase fraction means the tumor is more aggressive. Other tests that may be ordered to measure the rate of growth are **thymidine labeling index (TLI), mitotic activity index (MAI)** and **Ki67.** These tests measure cell proliferation and may also be referred to as **cell kinetics.**

- **Hormone Receptor Assay**—Hormone receptor assay is a test that measures the presence of estrogen (ER) and progesterone (PR) receptors in the tumor cell nuclei. It tells the physician whether the tumor was stimulated to grow by female hormones and is very important in determining what type of treatment will be used after surgery. If a tumor is positive, that means it was stimulated by estrogen or progesterone and usually carries a more positive prognosis.

- **Tumors May Be:**

  ER positive (+) PR positive (+)

  ER positive (+) PR negative (-)

  ER negative (-) PR positive (+)

  ER negative (-) PR negative (-)

- **Blood Vessel or Lymphatic Invasion**—A microscopic examination of the tumor will show if the surrounding blood vessels (vascular) or lymphatic vessels have been invaded by the tumor. No invasion offers a better prognosis.

- **HER2/neu**—A prognostic indicator that is over-expressed or amplified in about 25 to 30 percent of breast cancers. Elevation of HER2 indicates a more aggressive cancer. However, identification of elevation indicates that a drug called Herceptin®, which targets the HER2/neu receptor, is an appropriate treatment choice.

- **p53**—Determines elevation of oncogenes (substances within cells that promote tumor development) to predict potential recurrence.

- **Tumor necrosis**—Observes the death of cancer cells inside the tumor.

Triple Negative Breast Cancer

Recently, the term "triple negative" breast cancer has been used to describe a woman's cancer when tests for three different breast cancer receptors are all negative. A triple negative breast cancer is one that is negative for estrogen receptors (ER), progesterone receptors (PR) and HER2 receptors (human epidermal growth factor receptor 2). Many drugs used in cancer treatment are designed to target one of these positive receptor sites, thus a triple negative breast cancer diagnosis limits the use of some medications. Triple negative women, however, are typically responsive to chemotherapy drugs that are not targeted at ER/PR or HER2 receptor sites.

Final Pathology Report

There are many other diagnostic tests being used to evaluate tumors. The physician will discuss the tests selected to evaluate the patient's tumor. Each of these tests helps to collect pieces of the puzzle needed for the oncologist to determine the best treatment.

The pathologist prepares a written report that is sent to the patient's physician. Time varies as to when the final report will be available. The pathologist's findings help the physician determine which surgery and treatment will be needed. Further diagnostic tests, such as additional blood work, a bone scan, liver scan, chest X-ray, CT scan or an MRI (magnetic resonance imaging), may be ordered.

Breast Cancer Stages 0 – 4

When the results are received from the tests, the cancer will be **staged** on a scale from zero (in-situ cancer) to four (a cancer with distant metastasis). A stage zero cancer is the earliest form of breast cancer and has the best prognosis. Staging is an estimate of how much the cancer has spread and is important in the selection of appropriate treatment (refer to pages 124–125).

Breast Cancer Stages

STAGE 0

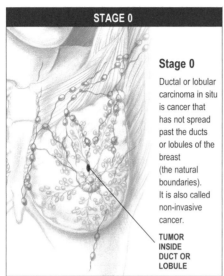

Stage 0

Ductal or lobular carcinoma in situ is cancer that has not spread past the ducts or lobules of the breast (the natural boundaries). It is also called non-invasive cancer.

TUMOR INSIDE DUCT OR LOBULE

STAGE 1

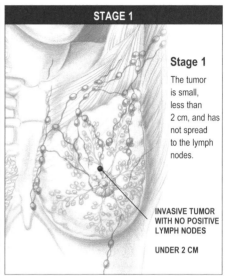

Stage 1

The tumor is small, less than 2 cm, and has not spread to the lymph nodes.

INVASIVE TUMOR WITH NO POSITIVE LYMPH NODES

UNDER 2 CM

STAGE 2

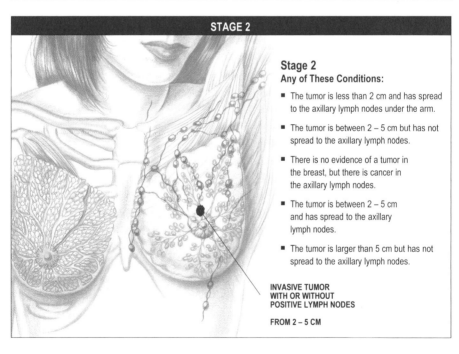

Stage 2
Any of These Conditions:

- The tumor is less than 2 cm and has spread to the axillary lymph nodes under the arm.

- The tumor is between 2 – 5 cm but has not spread to the axillary lymph nodes.

- There is no evidence of a tumor in the breast, but there is cancer in the axillary lymph nodes.

- The tumor is between 2 – 5 cm and has spread to the axillary lymph nodes.

- The tumor is larger than 5 cm but has not spread to the axillary lymph nodes.

INVASIVE TUMOR WITH OR WITHOUT POSITIVE LYMPH NODES

FROM 2 – 5 CM

Breast Cancer Stages

STAGE 3

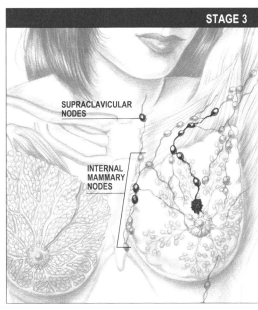

SUPRACLAVICULAR NODES

INTERNAL MAMMARY NODES

Stage 3
Any of These Conditions:

- The tumor is smaller than 5 cm and has spread to axillary lymph nodes that are attached to each other or to other structures.

- The tumor is larger than 5 cm and has spread to the axillary lymph nodes, which may or may not be attached to each other or to other structures.

- The tumor has spread to the chest wall, caused swelling or ulceration of the breast or is diagnosed as inflammatory breast cancer.

- The tumor (of any size) has not spread to distant parts of the body but has spread to the lymph nodes above the collarbone, under the collarbone or both the nodes inside the breast and the internal mammary nodes.

STAGE 4

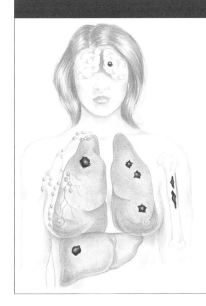

Stage 4
Distant Metastasis:

The tumor can be any size and has spread to other sites in the body, usually the bones, lungs, liver, brain or lymph nodes far from the breast.

Three Basic Factors Considered in Staging Are (TNM):

- **T**umor size (T)

- Lymph **N**ode involvement (N)

- **M**etastasis to other areas (M)

When the patient returns to the physician for the pathology results, the patient may want to ask the following questions and write down the answers. (Some doctors will provide a copy of the pathology report for her records, and some pathologists will be happy to talk with the patient.) Early in the diagnostic work-up, all of the answers to the following questions may not yet be available.

Pathology Report Questions:

- What is the name of the type of cancer she has?

- Was the tumor in situ (inside ducts or lobules) or infiltrating (invasive— grown through the duct or lobule walls into surrounding tissues)?

- What size was the tumor? (The size is in millimeters (mm) or centimeters (cm). 10 mm equal 1 cm. 1 cm equals ⅜ inch. 1 inch equals approximately 2.5 cm.)

- Was the cancer found anywhere else in her breast tissue?

    - **Multifocal:** means additional cancer was found in the same quadrant of the breast.

    - **Multicentric:** means that it was found in another quadrant of the breast distant from the tumor.

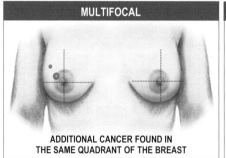

MULTIFOCAL

ADDITIONAL CANCER FOUND IN
THE SAME QUADRANT OF THE BREAST

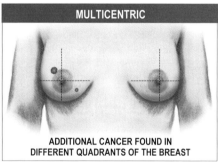

MULTICENTRIC

ADDITIONAL CANCER FOUND IN
DIFFERENT QUADRANTS OF THE BREAST

- How many lymph nodes were removed? Sentinel node biopsy alone usually removes from one to three nodes. (Approximately 75 percent of tumors have two sentinel nodes).

- How many levels of lymph nodes did you sample or remove? (There are three levels of nodes. Most axillary dissection removes levels one and two.)

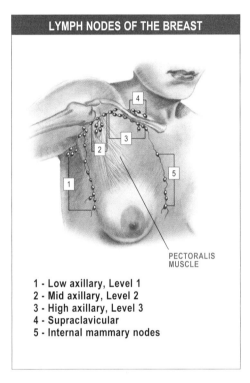

LYMPH NODES OF THE BREAST

PECTORALIS MUSCLE

1 - Low axillary, Level 1
2 - Mid axillary, Level 2
3 - High axillary, Level 3
4 - Supraclavicular
5 - Internal mammary nodes

- Were any nodes positive for cancer cells?

- Were the tumor receptors for estrogen or progesterone positive or negative?

- What was the cell proliferation status? (Indicator of how fast cancer is/ was growing at the time of surgery.)

- Was the tumor positive for HER2?

- Is there anything else that she needs to know about her cancer?

Major Pathology Factors

Reading a complete pathology report can be overwhelming because of all of the medical language. As a support partner, there are just a few major facts that you need to understand. The main components of the report that determine the patient's final treatment plan are the stage of the cancer, hormone receptor status, HER2 status, lymph nodes status and whether the cancer has metastasized to other parts of her body. If you have a copy of the pathology report, you can find these characteristics by looking for the answers to the following questions. If you are unable to identify these major facts, mark the characteristic and ask her physician to clarify the results. (Check the boxes that apply.)

Pathology Report Information:
1. Hormone receptor status
☐ ER positive (+) PR positive (+)

☐ ER positive (+) PR negative (-)

☐ ER negative (-) PR positive (+)

☐ ER negative (-) PR negative (-)

☐ Could not determine; ask doctor for test results

2. HER2 receptor status
☐ HER2 positive (HER2+)

☐ HER2 negative (HER2-)

☐ Could not determine; ask doctor for test results

3. Lymph node status
☐ Lymph node positive

☐ Lymph node negative

☐ Could not determine; ask doctor for test results

Surgical Information:

4. Stage of her cancer

☐ Stage 0

☐ Stage 1

☐ Stage 2

☐ Stage 3

☐ Stage 4

☐ Ask doctor for information

5. Has her cancer metastasized?

☐ Yes

☐ No

☐ Ask doctor for information

6. If yes, where has her breast cancer metastasized?

☐ Bones

☐ Lungs

☐ Liver

☐ Brain

☐ Other

☐ Ask doctor for information

Remember...

The pathology report contains information needed to determine treatment decisions.

Individuals must decide how much they wish to understand about their cancer.

As a support partner, it is most helpful if you assist her in getting the pathology report and understanding it to the degree that she feels comfortable.

Support Partner
Perspectives

"As a little league football coach, I learned that the first step to winning is to build a good team. I thought about this when my mate faced a breast cancer diagnosis. If we were to win this game, we needed the best team. Our family doctor acted as head coach, my wife became the quarterback, and, at times, I only felt like the water boy; but, by putting together the best medical and supportive team we could, we knew we were doing all that was humanly possible to give her the best chance for recovery."

—**Al Barrineau, Support Partner**

"Instead of complaining that she needed chemotherapy, she was grateful that there was something that could be done to treat her cancer—just like my mom to think this way! She didn't look forward to treatments; instead she looked forward to getting rid of any cancer that may have been left in her body after surgery."

—**Krystle Brown-Shaw, Support Partner**

CHAPTER 16

Treatments for Breast Cancer

After the final pathology report is studied, the oncologist (a physician who treats cancer) will recommend a plan of treatment. This may include chemotherapy (treatment with cancer-fighting drugs), radiation therapy (X-ray) or hormonal therapy. Medical oncologists specialize in treating patients with chemotherapy, and radiation oncologists specialize in radiation therapy. Some women may receive all of the treatment modalities. Others may receive only one type of treatment. Some may not receive any additional treatment because of their tumor characteristics and the surgery performed.

Oncologists carefully review the pathology report and any other tests, perform a thorough physical exam and then prescribe a treatment plan.

Treatment Plan Factors:
- Cancer cell type
- Tumor size
- In situ or invasive cancer
- Tumor growth rate or how much cells have changed from original cells (predictor of aggressiveness)
- Tumor markers (HER 2)
- Estrogen and progesterone hormone receptor status (positive or negative)
- Lymph node involvement (positive or negative)
- Cancer found in other parts of the body
- Menopausal state of the patient
- Medical history and general health of patient

Remember, there is more than one kind of breast cancer, and different types of cancers may require different treatments. Some types of cancer (inflammatory) and cancer that has spread to other parts of the body may require chemotherapy administration before surgery is performed (neo-adjuvant). Do not compare her treatment with another patient's because you will probably be comparing two entirely different cases because of breast cancer's wide variabilities in treatment.

Oncotype DX®

In the past several years, a new test, Oncotype DX, has become available for women with early stage breast cancer to predict the potential for recurrence and whether chemotherapy is likely to benefit a patient. The test analyzes 21 different genes in the tumor sample that are known to predict a higher rate of recurrence. This information helps oncologists and patients make more informed treatment decisions about chemotherapy based on a woman's individual cancer.

Criteria for Testing:
- Stage I and II cancer
- Estrogen (ER) receptor positive
- Negative (cancer-free) lymph nodes or have nodes showing micrometastases. Certain patients with cancer in only one to three lymph nodes may benefit from testing. Ask her physician.
- HER2 negative or equivocal status

Oncotype DX is not appropriate for women diagnosed with in situ (ductal or lobular) breast cancer or for women with later stage disease.

How The Test Is Performed
A pathology slide of the tumor that was removed during surgery (biopsy, lumpectomy or mastectomy) is shipped for testing. The physician (surgeon or oncologist) may order the test if the patient qualifies.

Oncotype DX Recurrence Score® Report
Test results are returned to the ordering physician with a Recurrence Score from 0 to 100. The Recurrence Score corresponds to the potential for breast cancer recurrence within a period of 10 years from the time of diagnosis and correlates with the likelihood of benefiting from chemotherapy. The lower the score, the lower the risk her cancer will recur. Women with low scores are also less likely to benefit from chemotherapy. It is important to

know that a lower Recurrence Score does not mean that there is no chance that breast cancer will return. The test analyzes the genes and serves as a prediction, not an absolute fact. It is based on the latest scientific methods known in determining cancer treatment appropriateness. Knowing the genomic profile of a cancer allows the physician to plan and tailor a treatment plan for the patient's cancer.

Chemotherapy

Chemotherapy drugs are usually given intravenously (through a vein), but occasionally they are administered by pill. Treatments usually consist of a combination of several drugs. They begin several weeks after final surgery and are given in a clinic or a physician's office. Frequency of administration may vary according to the treatment plan. Most treatments are given every three weeks. Recently the schedule for some patients has been shortened to a two-week interval and is called "dose-dense" chemotherapy. The same dose (amount) of chemotherapy may be administered every two weeks when drugs are given to support the blood cell's repopulation after chemotherapy administration, if needed. Side effects vary according to the drugs, amount of drugs administered and the individual patient. The treatment team will supply information on the drugs and on management of side effects.

Some women with veins that are difficult to find with an I.V. needle, or those who are to receive certain types of drugs, may require a permanent device inserted under the skin called a venous access device or a "port" ("port-a-cath").

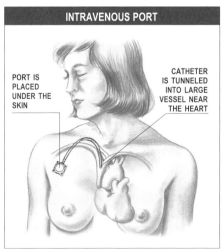

INTRAVENOUS PORT

PORT IS PLACED UNDER THE SKIN

CATHETER IS TUNNELED INTO LARGE VESSEL NEAR THE HEART

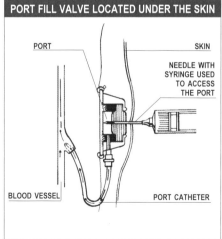

PORT FILL VALVE LOCATED UNDER THE SKIN

PORT

SKIN

NEEDLE WITH SYRINGE USED TO ACCESS THE PORT

BLOOD VESSEL

PORT CATHETER

This device is usually placed under the skin on the chest wall during a brief outpatient surgery and is used to administer chemotherapy and draw blood samples. This prevents the discomfort of numerous I.V. sticks during her period of treatment. The patient is able to perform normal activities with the device, including bathing and swimming.

Radiation Therapy

Radiation therapy is provided by a radiation oncologist, a physician specializing in the treatment of cancer using radiation. Radiation destroys microscopic cancer cells by making them unable to divide and multiply. When the cancer cells die, the body naturally eliminates them. Healthy cells are able to repair themselves in a way that cancer cells cannot. Radiation therapy is usually administered after a lumpectomy for six to seven weeks. It may also be used for local control to destroy any cancer cells when cancer has spread into an area. Radiation kills cells in only the area of treatment; whereas, chemotherapy acts systemically, killing cancer cells throughout the body.

Treatment usually begins when the surgical incision has healed, usually after four to six weeks, or it may be started at the completion of chemotherapy treatments. During the initial visit, the area is carefully marked for future treatment. Each treatment under the machine only takes minutes to deliver. However, the appointment time is usually about thirty minutes, allowing the patient time to undress, have a technologist check her records and set the adjustments on the machine. Treatments are given on a daily basis, Monday through Friday, ranging from six to seven weeks. Side effects are generally mild, but may include changes in the skin over the treated area similar to a mild sunburn, mild fatigue and, occasionally, a sore throat. The treatment team will provide information on the management of side effects.

Hormonal Therapy

Hormonal therapy may be recommended if the studies performed on the tumor prove to be positive for stimulation by estrogen (ER+) or progesterone (PR+). There are several major kinds of hormonal therapy. The decision of the appropriate drug will be based, in part, on whether a woman is pre- or postmenopausal. Some of the drugs lower the amount of estrogen in the body, some block estrogen receptors on the cells and some shut down the production of estrogen in the body.

Hormonal Drug Categories:

- **SERMs (Selective Estrogen-Receptor Modulators):** block the estrogen receptors on the cell so that estrogen cannot enter. The two drugs used are Nolvadex® (tamoxifen) and Evista® (raloxifene).

- **Aromatase inhibitors:** reduce the amount of estrogen the body produces in postmenopausal women. Three of the drugs are Arimidex® (anastrozole), Aromasin® (exemestane) and Femara® (letrozole).

- **ERDs (Estrogen-Receptor Down Regulators):** destroy the estrogen receptor on the cell. The drug currently in use is Faslodex® (fulvestrant). Ovarian shutdown or removal drugs are Zoladex® (goserelin acetate) and Lupron® (leuprolide), and they are given by injection once a month for several months.

Hormonal medication may be given in many different ways: alone, in combination or one after the other.

Breast Cancer Genetic Testing

In 1994 and 1995, two mutated (changed) genes, BRCA1 and BRCA2 (BR=breast, CA=cancer), were discovered. These genes cause 7 – 10 percent of breast cancers. A blood test can now determine if a person is a carrier of either of these mutated genes and the possible cause of her breast cancer. These two genes also cause a woman to be at high risk for ovarian cancer.

After a breast cancer diagnosis, the healthcare team can review the patient's family and personal history to determine if she meets the criteria for genetic testing. Breast or ovarian cancer in the history of either parent is also an important consideration. One important factor about genetic mutations is that they can be inherited from a mother or father. For years, only the mother's family history was considered to put a woman at higher risk. We now know that the risk comes equally from the father.

Genetic testing can determine if the patient has a mutation in either of these identified genes. If positive, her children, male or female, are at a 50 percent risk of inheriting these defective genes, which they can then pass on to their offspring. Having a mutated gene places them at higher risk for breast, ovarian or other cancers.

Criteria for BRCA1 or BRCA2 Testing:

- Diagnosed with either breast cancer before age 50 or ovarian cancer at any age
- Diagnosed with bilateral (both sides) breast cancer or have multiple primary sites of cancer
- Family history of male breast cancer
- Have a blood relative who is documented as being a BRCA mutation carrier
- Individuals of Ashkenazi Jewish descent with a personal or family history of breast cancer
- Have one first degree (mother, father, sister, brother, daughter or son) or second degree (aunt, uncle, grandparent, grandchild, niece, nephew, half-brother or half-sister) relative younger than 50 who was diagnosed with breast and/or ovarian cancer

Benefits of Testing:

- Allows the patient to know if her cancer was related to one of these mutated genes.
- A negative test, showing no gene mutation, means that the gene for breast cancer was not passed on to children of the patient. Prevents unnecessary anxiety about children being high risk and prevents future expensive surveillance tests.
- Positive test allows family members to choose to be tested or placed in high risk surveillance programs.
- Positive test may alter recommendations for future treatment of breast cancer and indicate a need for surveillance for ovarian cancer or prophylactic surgical removal of ovaries.

If there is a history of breast cancer or ovarian cancer on either side of the patient's family, discuss the benefits of genetic testing with a qualified healthcare provider. Testing consists of having a vial or syringe (several tablespoons) of blood drawn and sent to a laboratory for testing. It is suggested that the patient be counseled about the procedure before blood is drawn and tested, and after the test results are given.

For up-to-date information on genetic breast cancer, visit the Web site www.myriadtests.com.

Clinical Trials

Occasionally, as part of treatment decisions, some women may have the opportunity to participate in new treatments called clinical trials. These are new investigational studies that research effective treatment and prevention strategies. Thousands of research studies are currently underway in the United States. Most trials are conducted by the National Cancer Institute, major medical centers or pharmaceutical companies. If a new treatment is determined safe and effective at the completion of the trial, the U.S. Food and Drug Administration (FDA) grants approval for its widespread commercial use by patients.

Four Phases of Clinical Trials:

- **Phase I** trials test new treatments to determine the acceptable dose and administration method.

- **Phase II** trials study the safety and effectiveness of the drug and how it affects the human body.

- **Phase III** trials require that a large number of patients receive either the standard therapy or the newer therapy in order to compare beneficial survival results and quality of life during treatment. If the newer drug is found to be more effective than the standard one, the trial is stopped and all participants are eligible for the more successful treatment. If there is any evidence that the newer drug is inferior or has unusual toxic side effects, the experimental medication is discontinued.

- **Phase IV** trials are conducted to further evaluate long-term safety and effectiveness of the trial drug after approval for standard use.

Clinical Trial Informed Consent

The doctor or nurse will explain in detail the type and purpose of the trial. The patient will be given an informed consent form to read and sign. This form must include the expected benefits, the negative aspects, other treatment options, assurance that the patient's personal records will be kept confidential, the negative aspects and a statement indicating that her participation is voluntary and she may withdraw at any time.

Participating in the trial does not prevent her from getting any additional medical care she may need. If she decides to participate in the trial, she will need to contact her insurance provider to ask if it covers any financial charges. Be sure the researchers are aware if her plan does not cover the costs of clinical trials. Some trials are simply a comparison of two drugs or timing of administration to determine which is more effective. Your physician will explain the details of the trial.

Questions To Ask About Clinical Trials:

- What phase is the clinical trial now in? (Phase I, II, III or IV)

- Who is sponsoring the study? (Needs to be approved by a reputable national group like the National Cancer Institute, a major teaching institution or the FDA.)

- What is the purpose of this study?

- What advantage does this trial have compared to standard recommended treatment?

- How long will the clinical trial last?

- Where will treatments be given and evaluated while on the trial?

- Is the drug or combination of drugs available outside the clinical trial?

- How will the success of the treatment be evaluated? (Blood tests, scans, etc.)

- How much additional time will participating in the trial require over standard treatment?

- Will there be any extra expenses or will all costs of the trial be covered?

- Will her insurance company cover the cost of the trial?

- What type of follow-up will continue after the trial is completed?

Understanding Clinical Trials

If you want to know more about clinical trials, the most obvious place to start is with your oncologist. The Cancer Information Service (CIS), a program supported by the National Cancer Institute, can compile information about the latest nationwide cancer treatments for a specific type and stage of cancer. For more information on clinical trials, you can access the Physician's Data Query (PDQ). (www.cancer.gov/cancerinfo/pdq/cancerdatabase)

To Participate or Not To Participate

The decision to participate in a clinical trial is often not an easy one to make. This decision is very personal and one that can only be made after the patient has discussed the advantages and disadvantages with her physician and clinical trial nurse. You can best help by assisting her in getting her questions answered about participating in the trial. When the final decision is made, she needs to feel that she has chosen what is best for her. Some women prefer the "tried and true," while others feel that they are getting an even better chance by taking a newer drug or drug combination. Some feel that by their participation in clinical trials they will be helping other women in the future. Remember, no one has the right answer to the question of whether or not one should or should not participate; there is not an absolute answer. That is why it is called a "trial."

Remember...

Treatment is based on the final surgical pathology report and the individual characteristics of the patient to determine the need for chemotherapy, radiation therapy or hormonal therapy.

BRCA1 and BRCA2 genes are inherited genes that place a woman at extremely high risk for breast or ovarian cancer. Testing can identify those who carry a mutated gene.

Clinical trials are studies to determine more effective methods to treat disease. Whether or not to participate in a clinical trial is a choice some women may be asked to make.

Support Partner Perspectives

"*The one I loved most was battling for her life. We were in this together.*"

—**Al Barrineau, Support Partner**

"*After surgery, I told Mom she had to stop taking care of everyone else and take care of herself. So, I told her I was taking over...lots of laughs from a daughter's perspective here. I put my foot down and demanded that she start getting more rest. Somehow, I think this is what she needed to hear from me. She needed to know that this is what I wanted to do. We have always been there for each other, and this made no difference. What a gift to know that you can show someone how much you love them when they really need it.*"

—**Krystle Brown-Shaw, Support Partner**

Your Partnership in Recovery

The next phase of recovery for the patient and family begins when the patient returns home. The strong emotions experienced during the diagnostic and surgical period dissipate and are replaced with new, lower emotional tones and challenges. As the patient returns home from surgery, the conflict of merging new family roles with the old routines—meals, cleaning, laundry, jobs and school—becomes the focus. The patient often struggles with the realization that she may not be able to physically maintain her role in the family immediately after surgery or for periods of time during chemotherapy or radiation treatments. These changes may become challenging as family life takes on a more somber emotional tone and the focus changes to incorporating unplanned cancer treatments into the daily routine. This usually requires reassigning many of the chores of daily living she would normally perform to someone else for a period of time. As a support person, you can serve an invaluable role and strengthen your relationship with the patient by becoming a part of the solution and redistributing some of her routine chores.

Look for opportunities to help her physically, as well as emotionally. When she returns home, she will probably need to have her dressing changed and her drain bulbs emptied. Some women appreciate assistance, while others feel uncomfortable. Ask her how you, and the family, can be most helpful.

The treatment team will instruct her on when to begin an exercise program that will help her regain strength and mobility in her surgical arm. One patient's support partner became the "captain of her physical therapy team." The partner reminded her of her exercises and helped her perform them. By participating with her in the dull, routine exercise series, this partner restored a vital sense of caring in the patient's mind.

This teamwork during boring exercises kept them emotionally in touch during her time of physical readjustment.

If surgery is the only treatment the patient requires for her cancer, she should have her physical energy return to near normal in about six weeks. There may be some lingering strength limitations in the surgical arm, but the arm will improve as she regains her full range of motion from her exercises and resumes normal activities. She will continue to have occasional sensations in the incisional area such as shooting pain or aching as it continues to heal; this is normal. However, you will find her emotional recovery after the cancer diagnosis takes much longer than the physical recovery. We will discuss her emotional recovery in Chapter 20.

Support Partner Perspectives

"I do not like hospitals. I do not like being around sick people. But the person I loved most in the world was having to have chemotherapy treatments in our fight to save her life. I was glad to go with her."

—*Al Barrineau, Support Partner*

"The toughest times for me were when I saw Mom gradually losing her strength due to the side effects of treatments. I saw her body slowly grow weaker, her pace get slower and her mood become more solemn. What I did not see was her spirit 'giving up.' She always found something to be hopeful about, even if it was just having the strength to sit up and look out of the window on the days her body was weakened by treatments. Her body was weak, but her spirit and determination to fight remained strong."

—*Krystle Brown-Shaw, Support Partner*

Support During Chemotherapy and Radiation Therapy

Chemotherapy or radiation treatments are often required after surgery. For patients, the time of chemotherapy or radiation therapy can be very anxiety-provoking. While the patient will probably have physically recovered enough to go to her treatments alone, psychologically she may need someone to accompany her, especially on the first few visits. A support person—you, a family member or friend—can help relieve her anxiety and help her understand the oncologist's explanations about her treatments. She may be hesitant to ask for you to go with her, but she will be very grateful when you offer to go or find someone else to accompany her. Others may not want "so much fuss" made over their treatments and will feel more in control if they go alone when they are physically able. Communicating your willingness and desire to share this time is important to her.

Planning to be helpful during treatments begins by understanding what her treatments involve.

Treatment Questions:

- How often will treatments be administered?
- How long will each treatment session last?
- Is someone allowed to be with her during these treatments?
- What are the expected side effects of the treatment? When do they occur?
- Will any medication be given prior to, or after, treatments that could prevent her from driving?
- At what time during the treatment cycle will she become the most fatigued?
- At what time during the treatment cycle will she be most vulnerable to infections?
- Are there any side effects, signs or symptoms that need to be recognized and reported to the healthcare team?

By understanding these facts, you will be able to make this time as psychologically and physically comfortable as possible. Plan to prepare or have food available during treatment dates so she will not feel responsible for meals. She may wish to schedule chemotherapy treatments to be given on Fridays, so you can take over household responsibilities on the weekend, allowing her plenty of time to rest. One family made a ritual of renting several movies and made this their weekend to catch up on their movie watching. The children pulled their sleeping bags into the den, and everyone "camped out" around Mom. The weekend was eagerly anticipated by the family, instead of dreaded, despite the physical discomfort experienced by the patient. Carefully assess her physical and psychological needs so that you may be as supportive as possible during treatment.

The weeks between treatments may also require that her daily responsibilities be redistributed among family members, co-workers and friends. One husband told of his experience of taking on unaccustomed chores: *"I already did most of the cooking, but I learned to do the laundry, only ruining a few items as I learned. I must confess, I found out what causes pink underwear. We had a cleaning person come in one day a week on a regular basis. The expense was not too great and was certainly worth the energy it saved. Ideally, I wanted the kids to do more; however, they are normal and haven't become much more useful around the house."* Recognize the need for changes in household chores, family, work and community activities. Take the initiative in reassigning responsibilities and helping prioritize her duties during recovery.

Understanding the Side Effects of Chemotherapy

Chemotherapy kills the rapidly dividing cancer cells in the body. Unfortunately, it also kills other rapidly dividing cells—blood cells, hair cells and cells that line the intestinal track. Most bothersome side effects occur when chemotherapy damages these cells—nausea, vomiting, diarrhea, mouth sores, hair loss, potential for infection, increased potential for bleeding, etc. The good news is that most of these side effects are time-limited during chemotherapy, and medications are readily available to treat them when they occur.

Chemotherapy also impacts her body's hormones. Estrogen, progesterone and testosterone are greatly impacted, lowering them to levels that cause the noticeable side effects of menopause. These side effects include mood swings, hot flashes, night sweats, vaginal dryness and numerous other symptoms. Unlike other side effects, the effects of lowered hormones may linger well after treatment ends.

Chemotherapy treatments may impact a relationship both physically and emotionally. It is physically trying to undergo chemotherapy for the patient, and this has a ripple effect for the one supporting her. Emotionally, the stress of dealing with the changes that cancer treatment brings into a family can become challenging for both the patient and her support partner.

As a support partner, understanding the major side effects and knowing what you can do to help reduces some of the impact and greatly improves her quality of life. We will discuss the impact of fatigue, hair loss, weight gain, insomnia, hot flashes, night sweats, mood swings, urinary problems and vaginal dryness.

Fatigue From Chemotherapy

After a chemotherapy treatment, the patient's energy level will be low. She will not feel like doing much of anything for several days after the infusion of drugs. These are the days she will experience the most nausea, vomiting or diarrhea. These acute side effects subside, but usually mid-cycle between treatments is when the drugs lower her blood counts to the lowest level, causing her to feel the most fatigued and to be most susceptible to infections. This time is called the "nadir" of treatment—when the blood levels fall to their lowest levels from treatment. Fatigue will vary with the type of drugs she receives. Ask her physician about the drugs and expected levels of fatigue. Fatigue has a cumulative effect, increasing as treatment progresses. Encourage her to get additional rest by taking naps or sleeping in when possible. Reduce as many of the tasks of daily living as possible during highest levels of fatigue. Take the initiative to divide household responsibilities among family members or consider hiring help during this time. Most women are least fatigued the week before treatment. This is the time to plan activities requiring more energy. She may be physically and emotionally exhausted during treatment, but this is all temporary.

Be sure that her meals are nutritionally adequate; good nutrition is required to build new cells that replace those which chemotherapy destroys. She may be too tired to prepare nutritionally balanced meals and may need help in this area.

Treatments will end, blood counts will increase and energy will gradually return. It is important to know that the return of energy does not happen in days or weeks when treatment is completed, but requires months. Some women say that even a year passed before their normal, pre-treatment levels of energy returned.

Support Partner
Perspectives

"When my wife lost her hair during chemotherapy treatments, it was almost the proverbial 'straw that broke the camel's back.' Losing her hair seemed to strip her of the last defense she had in denial of her own cancer."

—**Al Barrineau, Support Partner**

"I wanted Anna to know that I, too, felt the emotional pain of her having to undergo treatment. When she had her first chemo treatment, I shaved my head, hoping in some way this would comfort her. I don't necessarily recommend this for others, but it helped me show her what I couldn't say. ... I tried to make getting better the only thing she had to worry about during her treatment. This was one thing I could 'fix' for her."

—**Brian Cluxton, Support Partner**

Hair Loss—The Most Painful Side Effect

Many women have expressed that the loss of their hair through chemotherapy treatments was the most distressing of all losses during breast cancer. Even though the loss is temporary, and the hair returns after treatment is completed, women have described its impact as *"being more upsetting than the loss of my breast."* Hair loss is difficult because it is outward evidence of the cancer process. It is often the first visible public display of their battle with cancer. It is much easier to camouflage the loss or alteration of a breast under clothing than the loss of hair with a wig.

The amount and timing of hair loss will vary according to the kind of drugs, the dosage of the drugs and the individual response to the drugs given. Most hair loss occurs between two and four weeks after the first treatment. Some treatment regimens will only cause gradual hair thinning; others will cause complete hair loss. To help her prepare for this occurrence in the treatment process, discuss with the treatment team how much hair loss she can expect and when it will most likely occur.

HAIR LOSS

When women in a focus group who had complete hair loss (alopecia) were asked to rate their emotional reactions to losing their hair:

- 50% reported it as severely emotionally painful

- 42% reported it as moderately emotionally painful

- 8% reported no emotional impact

When participants were asked to distinguish which was more emotionally distressing, their altered body image as a result of surgery, or hair loss, 74% reported hair loss as being the more emotionally painful.

To help her deal with hair loss, assure her of your total acceptance. Some women, knowing they will have hair loss, opt to have their hair cut short to help with the transition. It is recommended that she shop for a wig before she loses her hair to better match her hair color and style. Her wig will probably not be noticeable except to those who know she has lost her hair. Do not complain about the cost of a wig or insist on her getting one that she does not feel comfortable wearing. Support and understanding during this extremely sensitive time are very important for her emotional well-being.

Obviously, the day or week she loses her hair will be one of her lowest times emotionally. It is important to remember that you can't change it. You can't make things different. Your best response is your reassuring presence. Allow her to grieve her loss and shed tears as much as she feels is necessary. At this time, there seem to be no good words that can bring comfort equal to the pain she feels.

Some people revert to jokes and humor during uncomfortable and painful times. However, refrain from using nicknames such as "Baldie," "Kojak" or other terms denoting hair loss. She may laugh outwardly but may inwardly feel differently. Let her take the lead in how she can best react to and manage her new appearance. Respect her privacy as she dresses and undresses. For some, it may be more difficult to allow you to see her bald head than to let you see her scar. Remember, hair loss is usually temporary. Therefore, don't insist that she show you her bald head or thinning hair if she feels uncomfortable. This will pass, unlike the change in her body image from surgery.

Some women will cling to the security of their wigs after their hair begins to return. She may need your encouragement to shed the wig and show off her new, shorter haircut. For some, this takes courage because they may have entered treatment with longer hair and may only feel comfortable returning to that image. This can be especially difficult if they feel that longer hair was important to you. Let her know of your acceptance early in the treatment phase.

Weight Gain After Treatment

Many women gain weight during and after breast cancer treatment. According to medical clinicians, reasons for weight gain include decreased activity with increased caloric intake, fluid retention from drugs, and effects on body metabolism from hormonal drugs and chemotherapy-induced menopause. Most women report that it was as if their metabolism changed overnight after treatment. They experienced weight gain even with the same amount of caloric intake as before. Even with an increase in physical activity after the treatment, their weight did not drop to pretreatment levels.

Weight gain is another potential obstacle for some women regarding their self-esteem. As you can tell from the focus group (see chart on page 149), 89 percent of women said weight gain had an impact on physical and sexual self-perception. As a supportive partner, remind her that weight gain is not necessarily a lack of self-control but a change of normal body metabolism. This reminder will help lay the foundation for her acceptance. We live in a culture where we are constantly told that a slim body is the desired norm for attractiveness. For many women, this is a very difficult change to deal with. Expressing your understanding, if she does gain weight, is a way to remove a recovery obstacle.

WEIGHT GAIN

54% of the participants reported gaining weight during or after treatment.

Those who gained weight were asked if they felt it affected their self-image and eventually had an effect on their sexual relationships:

- 53% said it had an impact on their sexual relationship

- 36% said it had some impact on their sexual relationship

- 11% said it had no impact on their sexual relationship

One way to help her is by encouraging her to get regular physical exercise. Suggest a regular physical activity together or as a family to have a regular time to share with each other (not so that she will lose weight, but for her overall health). The major focus should always be on good health, not her weight.

Insomnia

Most women have problems sleeping all night, starting when they find an abnormality in their breast, throughout treatment and well into recovery. Insomnia can be a continuing problem for women who take chemotherapy and remain in a menopausal condition.

The inability to sleep all night can contribute to fatigue, irritability, mental fogginess and depression. This often becomes like the chicken and egg debate: which comes first—these symptoms or insomnia? The appropriate answer is that whatever the cause, insomnia should be addressed and interventions offered by a healthcare provider. Insomnia should not be experienced week after week and dismissed as normal and unimportant. Chronic insomnia needs treatment; a night or two of interrupted sleep can be tolerated, but continued insomnia can cause grave coping and quality of life problems.

INSOMNIA

Data from the focus groups indicated that:

- 88% experienced insomnia during treatment

- 70% experienced insomnia six months after treatment

- 60% still suffered a year after treatment had ended

During interviews in the focus groups with women experiencing insomnia, the severity of sleeplessness correlated closely with the level of stress they were under (highest during diagnostic and early treatment phases). High levels of stress are naturally expected during a cancer diagnosis. For women who are regularly not sleeping all night because of stress, medications can greatly reduce insomnia. Sleeping medications are recommended for short-term use and are appropriate for a limited time. However, many women complain of continued drowsiness the next day and find that other options offer nearer to normal functioning the next day. Anti-anxiety medications are an option that relieve stress and allow her to sleep. Benadryl®, an over-the-counter antihistamine, is a safe sedative for most people and is found in medications like Tylenol PM®. Encourage her to contact her physician for recommendations or medications to help with her lack of sleep.

Hot Flashes and Night Sweats

For women who take chemotherapy, insomnia may be increased significantly in relation to the number of hot flashes and night sweats experienced. For these women, asking their healthcare provider for interventions to reduce hot flashes and night sweats is essential. Due to hot flashes, one woman in the focus group had not slept longer than two or three hours a night since her treatment had ended two years earlier. This is unacceptable. Hot flashes or night sweats that cause waking deserve attention from the healthcare team.

Hot flashes are the side effect from treatment that is most often reported to physicians. Hot flashes can be reduced greatly for most women by taking an SSRI (Selective Serotonin Reuptake Inhibitor) such as Effexor®, Paxil®, Prozac®, Celexa®, Zoloft®, Lexapro® or Luvox®. These drugs also assist with reducing depression and insomnia. For hot flashes or night sweats that do not respond to these interventions, a blood pressure medication, Catapres® (clonidine), has proven helpful for many women suffering severe symptoms. A combination of medications can reduce symptoms of insomnia, hot flashes and night sweats to a manageable level. It is important to consider quality of life issues and to understand that they need and deserve attention from her healthcare provider. This may mean changing providers to find one that addresses all issues, not just her cancer.

HOT FLASHES					
Hot Flashes	None	1 – 2 a Day	3 – 5 a Day	6 – 10 a Day	Over 10 a Day
Before Diagnosis	81%	10%	8%	0%	0%
During Treatment	32%	19%	25%	11%	13%
6 Months After Treatment	12%	26%	32%	13%	17%
12 Months After Treatment	14%	25%	27%	20%	14%

NIGHT SWEATS					
Night Sweats	None	1 – 2 a Day	3 – 5 a Day	6 – 10 a Day	Over 10 a Day
Before Diagnosis	75%	22%	3%	0%	0%
During Treatment	33%	25%	29%	9%	6%
6 Months After Treatment	25%	28%	36%	7%	4%
12 Months After Treatment	26%	42%	17%	9%	5%

Mood Swings

When women lose their estrogen, through natural or chemical menopause, one of the first things they notice is a change in their emotions. Before menopause, this is experienced the few days before their menstrual period and referred to as premenstrual syndrome (PMS). PMS occurs when estrogen and progesterone fall to their lowest levels to allow menstruation. During these few days, increased moodiness, tearfulness, nervousness and outbursts of anger are common symptoms in many women. The same symptoms occur during reduction of female hormones from chemotherapy. A sad fact is that women are often made to feel that their unstable emotions are caused because they are not "handling cancer" well or because they are depressed. The fact is, their bodies are thrown into the same emotional limbo as PMS, but it remains day after day because the hormones do not return to reverse the withdrawal. This emotional roller coaster is caused by the chemotherapy drugs and not the patient's emotional weakness or ability to "handle cancer".

It is almost a certainty that mood changes will occur during treatments. The reduction of the female hormones caused by treatment may cause wide fluctuations in the patient's moods. She may swing from normal to sad, then to angry, then to depressed—all with no apparent cause. It is important to understand that she, like you, dislikes the changes she experiences. Relate to her mood swings in an understanding manner, realizing the cause and not interpreting this as a sign of a diminishing relationship.

MOOD SWINGS
Participants in focus groups reported an increase in emotional mood swings:
■ 55% increase during treatment
■ 42% increase six months after treatment ended
■ 19% increase at one year after completing treatment
Mood changes after chemotherapy are an expected side effect and vary in degrees of intensity.

Urinary Problems

When estrogen levels are reduced, another common side effect is urinary symptoms. Estrogen receptors are found in the lining of the urinary bladder and tubes. When estrogen levels are low, the lining becomes thinner and some women experience burning during urination, urinary urgency and urinary stress incontinence (loss of urine when walking fast, running or sneezing). They find holding their urine difficult and often a source of embarrassment. There are interventions to reduce this side effect. The use of estrogen vaginal cream or Estring® will greatly reduce these symptoms. However, many physicians prefer to wait to treat this symptom until after cancer treatment has ended to avoid interfering with treatment medications.

Vaginal Dryness and Itching

Vaginal dryness is another side effect caused by estrogen reduction from chemotherapy or hormonal therapy. Vaginal dryness is not only uncomfortable, but it can also cause itching. The dryness of the vaginal tissues can set up an environment for irritating or painful vaginal infections that interfere with sexual pleasure. Any itching or swelling should be reported to the healthcare team for a vaginal infection evaluation. Infections may be caused by an overgrowth of bacteria that causes a thin, gray discharge that has a fishy odor. A fungus (Candida albicans) normally found in the body can experience an overgrowth (often caused by antibiotics) causing a discharge of thick, white (cottage cheese-like) clumps that cause itching along with internal and external swelling. Both of these vaginal infections can easily be treated with medications prescribed by her physician.

What Women Can Do About Vaginal Dryness

During natural menopause, women are offered oral or transdermal (patch applied to skin) hormone replacement therapy to relieve their symptoms. At this time, this is usually not an option during breast cancer treatment. However, after treatment is completed, if the vaginal dryness continues even though vaginal moisturizers and lubricants are used, encourage her to discuss other options with her healthcare provider. The first option would be estrogen vaginal cream applied inside the vagina and on the external vaginal lips, or Vagifem®, an estrogen tablet that is inserted into the vagina. Another option is a vaginal ring of estradiol (Estring®) that is inserted into the vagina and remains in place for three months, slowly releasing the drug before replacement is needed. These localized estrogens relieve vaginal dryness and decrease urinary symptoms. After several months, the vagina increases in moisture and elasticity, making intercourse far more comfortable.

Reducing Fatigue

Fatigue, as previously mentioned, is the most common symptom experienced during and after cancer treatment. It is an expected side effect, but one that also has interventions that can reduce its impact. To reduce fatigue, it is first necessary to manage other side effects, such as nausea and vomiting, diarrhea, hot flashes and insomnia, because they all contribute to increasing fatigue. The good news is that physical activity can also help to reduce fatigue.

Physical Activity as a Fatigue Intervention

Studies now show that physical activity can increase physical stamina and reduce many treatment side effects. People who have not participated in regular exercise think of exercise as an additional activity that will decrease their available energy and cause increased fatigue. The opposite is true. Physical exercise has proven to restore energy and reduce many side effects during cancer treatment and recovery.

Normal fatigue is expected after surgery, radiation therapy and chemotherapy. In the past the traditional recommendation was "you need to rest," and many patients reverted to bed rest to manage their fatigue. It was believed that the more one rested, the more quickly one would recover. However, newer studies have shown that too much bed rest can actually promote physiological changes that increase, rather than decrease, fatigue.

Studies by Greenleaf and Kozlowski revealed, *"Maintenance of optimal health in a person requires a proper balance between exercise, rest, and sleep, as well as time in an upright position."*

Bed Rest Versus Activity Study Revealed:

- Too **much** rest promotes fatigue (imbalance).

- Too **little** activity promotes fatigue (imbalance).

- A dynamic **balance** between rest and activity decreases fatigue.

Their conclusion was that patients need to remain as active as possible during periods of physical recovery. There has to be a balance of activity and rest for maximum energy to be maintained.

New Approach to Fatigue Management:

- Too much rest can decrease available energy.

- Exercise can build energy.

- Excessive bed rest and inactivity are enemies of recovery.

- Too much rest can cause increased fatigue and make a person feel worse.

- Activity and rest must be balanced to maintain or build energy.

- Maintaining or starting a moderate exercise program based on one's present ability can speed recovery and reduce symptoms of treatment; it will not be harmful.

- Exercise activities can reduce the need for pain and nausea medications that have side effects of fatigue.

With the new information available, this is an opportunity to help make her recovery a time of balance between appropriate rest and appropriate exercise. If she did not participate in an exercise activity prior to her cancer diagnosis, now is the time to encourage her to build energy by adopting moderate physical movement as a part of her complete recovery plan.

Whatever exercise she selects and consistently does will raise her energy levels and speed her psychological recovery from breast cancer by decreasing depression. In addition, exercise reduces pain by promoting the release of natural painkillers referred to as "endorphins" or "natural morphine" into the body.

Physical Activity Planning

Before beginning any exercise program, the patient should ask her physician if she has any limitations. While it is important to maintain physical activity, it is also necessary to understand that her tolerated level of activity may change during different phases of treatment. The goal is to strive to maintain physical activity at a level that allows her to exercise regularly without exhaustion.

Encourage her to incorporate a regular physical exercise program into her recovery. This is an area where a support partner can become an active participant by joining her in an activity that she enjoys. The rewards will be increased physical stamina, psychological well-being and a closer relationship.

What Type of Exercise Program Is Best?

The right exercise is something she can physically do, has the time to do, is convenient and she enjoys. She does not need to join a gym or health club. Walking programs, Pilates, yoga, biking, swimming or gardening are all good choices.

Starting a regular walking program is a good choice because it can be done at anytime she chooses, it does not cost anything and it can be adapted to her present physical condition. A walking program can be easily modified to meet her changing needs during treatment; it can be started, suspended, decreased or accelerated according to her physical energy.

Exercise Evaluation

The ultimate test to evaluate whether she is overdoing exercise is to wait one hour after completion and then ask her, *"Do you have more energy and feel more relaxed?"* If the answer is yes, she is exercising in a range that is building energy. If the answer is no, she is over-taxing her body's physical reserves, and she needs to reduce the intensity or duration of the exercise.

Suspend Exercise if She Has:

- Fever
- Nausea or vomiting
- Muscle or joint pain with swelling
- Bleeding from any source
- Irregular heart beat

- Dizziness or fainting
- Chest, arm or jaw pain
- Intravenous chemotherapy administration on the same day
- Blood drawing on the same day—may exercise afterwards, but prior exercise may alter counts
- Any restrictions placed on exercise activities by a physician
- Blood counts are at low levels
  - White blood count less than 3,000 mcL
  - Absolute granulocyte count less than 2,500 mm³
  - Hemoglobin/hematocrit less than 10 g/dL
  - Platelet count less than 25,000 mcL

Diet and Exercise

Diet and regular physical exercise can significantly improve how a patient will feel during treatment and recovery. Eating nutritious food and getting regular exercise are keys to increasing energy and improving mood. When the body has nutrients from food available and the ability to transport oxygen to all of its cells increased by regular exercise, it increases its capacity to heal, increases available energy, elevates mood, decreases pain, lowers anxiety, decreases depression and boosts immunity. The good news is that there is no prescription required.

As a support partner, these are two areas where you can be of encouragement. However, it is important not to push for change if she is resistant. Share your commitment to join her in these endeavors.

*R*emember...

Hair loss can be the most traumatic of all events for a breast cancer patient.

Chronic insomnia, night sweats and hot flashes can seriously impair quality of life and coping capabilities.

Encourage her to start a regular exercise activity to increase her energy and reduce fatigue.

Take Cancer One Day At A Time

As you begin your journey as a support partner
for the one you love with cancer,
take it one day at a time.

Don't spend too much time looking at the past and wondering "why,"
and don't look too far into the future asking "what."
Know that life can only be lived today.

Yesterday is history, tomorrow is the future,
and both are out of reach.
Today is the present, and the only time you can hold on to.

When the days are emotionally tough,
just know there are people who care about you
and are there to help.
Don't be too hard or expect too much of yourself.
Being a support partner is a new experience,
and there is much to learn.

Believe that if you take it one day at a time,
you can successfully fight your fears, self-doubt and emotional pain.
With prayer, humor, friends and your faith,
you can, as you have in the past,
move through this problem with courage.

You can then share the courage you find with the one you love.
Together, the two of you can walk through the journey of
breast cancer with hearts entwined,
holding hands while sharing each other's grief.

That's what being a support partner is all about.
Just take cancer one day at a time.

Judy Kneece

Support Partner
Perspectives

"*Sex was a difficult subject for me. I didn't want to make sexual advances, nor did I want Anna to think that she was not still as beautiful, sexy and desirable to me as before. I didn't want to put any pressure on her. I finally expressed my reservations and we talked through the issues. This helped both of us greatly.*"

—**Brian Cluxton, Support Partner**

"*We were both emotionally drained. I had to give my mate a chance to regroup. The actual sexual act could wait. However, we both needed touching, cuddling and holding each other. It was important that I tell her I still found her attractive. I allowed her to set the guidelines on how and when the sexual relationship would be resumed. … I was so grateful a surgical procedure could be performed to rid her body of the cancer. However, my mate had to make peace with her scar before she allowed me to see it. This took several days. We had been able to communicate about it from the beginning, and that helped us both. I was prepared for the scar and new body shape to be much worse than it was. I really didn't mind the way she looked. Her breast did not make her the person I loved, and the loss of her breast would not stop my loving her. The scar seemed easier for me to accept than for her—but then, it was her body that was involved and not mine. She needed my assurance that this would not change our relationship.*"

—**Al Barrineau, Support Partner**

CHAPTER 18

Sexuality After Breast Cancer

"After treatment, my husband felt very rejected because I had no desire for sex and was unable to respond to him sexually. This caused a lot of stress and negative feelings for three years. I kept asking my doctors for help, but to no avail. My husband and I finally sat down and discussed everything. I then went to a new OB/GYN and once again asked for help. Thank goodness, she helped us solve our problem with various interventions. Today we have a very good sexual relationship, but we missed out on at least three years due to lack of knowledge about what we could do. I don't believe either of us would have opted to skip chemo just for me to be sexually responsive. But it would have been very helpful to know what to expect before chemo and then to get help dealing with the side effects without having to wait three years."

—EduCare Focus Group Participant

Sexuality issues after breast cancer are the least discussed of all breast cancer issues. Yet sexuality issues can pose some of the greatest challenges for a patient and her sexual partner. The purpose of this chapter is to help support partners who have an intimate relationship with a patient understand the impact of chemotherapy on her sexual functioning. Our goal is to help you and your partner understand, adjust and prevent sexuality issues from becoming a roadblock to complete recovery.

The data used in this chapter is from national focus groups conducted by EduCare in hospitals to gather information about chemotherapy's impact on a breast cancer patient's sexual functioning.

FOCUS GROUPS

EduCare Inc. conducted research during 2000 and 2001 on sexuality after breast cancer treatment in focus groups of breast cancer survivors. The groups were convened in 11 different hospitals nationally. The purpose of the groups was to gather information from women who had taken chemotherapy about the impact it had on their sexual functioning and quality of life. Investigated were the physical changes experienced, the sexual changes, the impact on the relationship with their sexual partner, their educational needs before treatment and the women's request for future services of pre-treatment education and support to be offered by their healthcare team and facility.

Judy C. Kneece, RN, OCN, conducted the focus groups, with patients invited from their healthcare facilities, which hosted the groups. Groups were held in the southeast, northeast, midwest and southwest. A total of 126 survivors responded to 143 questions using individual Audience Response Interactive data pads. These hand-held computer pads allowed all answers to be anonymous. Each woman was free to express her true feelings without anyone knowing how she answered. The computer automatically analyzed the data entered at each individual site and then combined the 11 sites for the final analysis. Included throughout this book are portions of the data gathered.

Sexuality—An Almost Taboo Topic

Sexuality issues greatly impact a woman; however, the topic is almost a taboo topic by healthcare providers as part of patient teaching on side effects she can expect. Of the 126 women in the focus groups who had chemotherapy after their surgery, only 13 percent had any type of pretreatment discussion with anyone on their healthcare team about any potential side effects they could experience from chemotherapy. This left an overwhelming 87 percent who were not forewarned of the potential for sexual dysfunction from chemotherapy treatments. After treatment started, only an additional 5 percent had a healthcare provider discuss sexual issues. This meant that a large majority, 82 percent of women and their sexual partners, were left to discover the changes that would occur from chemotherapy treatment by themselves and to find ways to deal with these changes on their own.

SEXUAL EDUCATION

- Of the 18% of women who had discussions with healthcare providers about sexuality issues, the average length of time ranged from 2 – 4 minutes, revealing how little emphasis is placed on sexuality. When these women rated their discussion value on a scale of 1 (not helpful) to 10 (very helpful), they rated the value of the discussion at 6.4, or of moderate help to the issues they faced.

- When asked if they questioned a physician/nurse about their sexual functioning during treatment, 32% responded yes. However, 100% reported having questions or problems. Those who asked questions rated the information provided by their healthcare providers a 4.1, slightly less than somewhat helpful. When asked if a suggested intervention was effective, the respondents rated the helpfulness of the intervention recommended by a physician/nurse a mere 3.9.

- Participants were asked, *"How important do you think it is for a physician or nurse to discuss and offer suggestions about potential sexuality changes?"* On a scale of 1 to 10, the group rated the need at a whopping 9.4. When asked about the need for healthcare providers to give written information about dealing with sexuality changes, they rated the need for written information at 9.4.

- When asked the question, *"Would you have found it helpful for the physician/ nurse to have included your partner in this sexuality discussion?"*, the response received an 8.9 rating on a scale from 1 to 10. Further clarification of this response came when the participants were asked, *"Did you feel that your partner understood the multitude of changes you were experiencing during treatment that impacted your sexuality?"* The question received a 5.3 rating, indicating the partner only somewhat understood.

Patients Want Partners To Understand

The vast majority of focus group attendees, 89 percent, wanted their partners to understand what they were facing by having their healthcare provider discuss the topic with them. They often expressed that they did not understand the changes themselves and found it difficult to explain to their partner the changes they were undergoing. About half, 53 percent, reported that they felt their partners did not fully understand their struggles. Our goal is to help reduce problems in your relationship that come from a lack of understanding of the sexuality changes that occur after breast cancer treatment.

Communication About Sexuality

The first and major recommendation for sexual adjustment after breast cancer is to open communication between the patient, yourself and the healthcare team. This is where problem solving begins, and it should begin early. With information, you can anticipate changes and be prepared to deal with them emotionally and physically.

Often, when patients complain to their healthcare provider about sexuality issues, their complaints are taken lightly, which may cause the patient to think that sexuality issues are not important. They often stop asking or complaining and suffer in silence. Women deserve to have sexuality issues addressed as aggressively as pain, nausea or vomiting. All of these are quality of life issues. Encourage your partner to discuss problems with her healthcare team and ask for written information. Contact the organizations listed in the resource section of this book for additional information.

Surgical Impact on Sexuality

You may notice during the surgical period when the stress is overwhelming for both of you that sexual interests are diminished; this is normal. However, during periods of stress, the need for emotional closeness increases. Most women express that they really need and want more touching, hugging and emotional closeness during this stressful period; but they often don't know how to express this or are afraid to ask. You may also feel unsure about how to respond and find yourself withdrawing. Do not allow walls of silence and emotional isolation to separate you from your partner and diminish your physical closeness during this time because you are not sure how to treat her. Let her know you still desire to be close and to touch without sexual expectations or demands. Tell her that you would like for her to take the lead in letting you know when she is emotionally and physically ready to resume physical intercourse.

For years, the literature has indicated that the major sexual obstacle after breast cancer is the changed body image women experience from surgery. However, it seems not to be the major cause for most women. Approximately 50 percent of all breast surgeries are lumpectomy procedures, causing little alteration in physical self-image. Mastectomy patients are having reconstruction at higher rates to restore their body image, unlike women years ago who only had access to a prosthesis to restore their body image. No matter which surgery is chosen, lumpectomy, mastectomy or reconstruction, the surgical scar and the new body image will need to be addressed.

As previously discussed, one of the potential roadblocks to restoring the sexual relationship may be viewing the surgical scar area. If a woman accepts her new body image and, more importantly, feels that you do, the sexual relationship suffers only temporary effects. There is no future impact on sexual functioning after the stress and fatigue from surgery are over.

VIEWING THE SCAR

- When focus group members were asked how long it was before their partners viewed their changed body images, 75% replied that it was within days after surgery.

- When asked how they perceived their partners' response when viewing the scar for the first time:

    - 80% reported their partners were accepting and supportive.

    - 15% reported a neutral response.

    - 6% reported that they perceived their response as negative.

- 6% of women in these focus groups reported that their partners had never seen their scar. These women were still dressing and undressing behind closed doors or in the dark.

What may change during the post surgical period is how she feels about herself and how she views her attractiveness to you as a sexual partner. You must let her hear and be assured that her reshaped body image has not changed how you see her—that her true beauty, sexuality and attractiveness are just as strong for you now as they were before her surgery. This is essential for the normal resumption of the sexual relationship.

Although it may sound silly, it is important to know that cancer cannot be "caught" from a partner during the sexual relationship. There is no reason that a sexual relationship should not continue in the same manner as before the cancer diagnosis.

When can you resume intercourse after breast cancer surgery? As soon as the two of you feel you would like to. If no complications arise, the incision should heal in about four weeks following surgery. However, you may resume your sexual relationship before the area is totally healed. The best time to continue is when you both feel ready.

The surgical scar area will naturally be sore or sensitive, but your partner can lead you in how to prevent pain by altering positions to avoid pressure on the area. Be open in asking her if she has problems with you touching her surgical breast now or in the future. Some women express that the breast is sensitive and prefer it not to be touched or stroked. Others express the opposite feeling; they view their partner's avoidance of touching or stroking their surgical breast as a sign of rejection or non-acceptance of their new image. This creates a problem for partners. The only way you can solve this dilemma in your relationship is to ask her what she desires in the area of touch. You may even find that her desires for touching her breast may change, especially after sensitivity is diminished. The best advice for a good relationship is continued communication about the subject.

Viewing the Surgical Scar

Because viewing the surgical scar can be a roadblock to restoring an intimate physical relationship, planning before surgery to view the scar together as early as possible removes this potential barrier. For some, it will never be easy. Talking about it before surgery and planning together helps start the recovery process.

Deciding, in advance, to view the incision when the physician changes the dressing works well for many couples. The physician is there to answer any questions and explain how the scar will change as it heals. As a support partner, it is also helpful to watch as a nurse applies a new dressing, in case a dressing would need to be changed at home. It is very difficult to change a dressing on her own chest. This is a task that a support partner can perform that will be helpful. It also serves to promote the growth of acceptance and emotional bonding as a couple.

If your partner is having difficulty allowing you to see her new body image, don't force the issue of when, but encourage her to allow you to share this as soon as she feels she is able. Nudity after breast surgery is a difficult issue for many women. This event may threaten an intimate relationship more than any other aspect of the breast cancer experience. In fact, there are some women who have never allowed their partner to see them nude after surgery. Some women are still dressing and undressing in the dark or behind closed doors twenty years after surgery. With the passing of time, it never became emotionally easier to share their new body image with their partner.

Dr. Charles Carver, a professor of psychology at the University of Miami in Florida, conducted a study of 240 breast cancer surgical patients involved in long-term relationships and the surgery's impact on their relationships with their partners. Couples were followed for one year after surgery. Data from the study reported, *"How a husband reacts to his wife's breast cancer scars can have a big impact on her sense of femininity and the overall health of the couple's relationship. The less breast cancer patients felt their partners were bothered by their surgical scars, the more likely they were to report feeling feminine and attractive."*

One woman fondly recalled, *"He looked at my scar and said, 'This will always serve as our reminder of how lucky we were to be spared your life. … Your breast for your life. Thank God it was a breast and I still have you. What a deal!' Later, as I looked at my scar, I remembered what he had said, and it was easier for me to accept."* Giving special meaning to the new scar early helped this couple avoid a potential problem.

Dr. Carver concluded from the study, *"Overall, the more the women saw their partners as affectionate and emotionally involved after the surgery, the more satisfied they were with the relationship."*

Impact of First Sexual Encounter After Surgery

Dr. Carver's study also revealed this about the first sexual encounter after surgery: *"The higher women rated the quality of their first sexual experience after surgery, the greater their feelings of femininity and attractiveness, the less emotional distress they experienced and the more satisfied with their future relationship."* Women also reported that their perception of their sexual desirability to their partner came primarily from their partner expressing interest and initiating sex and the frequency of the sexual contact.

Radiation Therapy Impact on Sexuality

Radiation therapy to the breast area ranges from six to seven weeks of daily treatment (Monday through Friday). If the patient is not getting chemotherapy, radiation starts about four weeks after breast surgery, or when the incision is healed. If she is having chemotherapy, radiation usually follows chemotherapy.

During radiation treatments, your partner is not radioactive, and sexual contact can continue. However, you may notice that she may experience increased fatigue during treatments, resulting in diminished sexual interest. There are no lasting impacts on the sexual relationship from radiation therapy. The problem of continued fatigue is mainly a side effect of chemotherapy.

The side effects of radiation therapy to the breast are redness and tenderness, much like a slight sunburn. The breast may swell slightly (edema) during therapy, but this usually diminishes over several months to a year after treatment. The patient may feel less sensitivity in the breast when touched and may notice that the skin of the breast feels slightly increased in thickness. The entire breast may feel firmer, with the skin appearing slightly tanned.

Chemotherapy Impact on Sexuality

If chemotherapy is required, sexuality changes become a more long-term challenge because of the impact of the drugs. Most chemotherapy patient teaching is about the well-known side effects of fatigue, nausea, vomiting and hair loss. Very few couples are forewarned about the impact on their sexual functioning, other than the potential for infertility if the woman is premenopausal. The main problem is that chemotherapy most often causes instant menopause in premenopausal women and increases menopausal side effects for menopausal women. Menopausal symptoms include hot flashes, night sweats, mood swings, irritability, vaginal dryness, painful intercourse, insomnia and numerous other changes.

Menopause caused by chemotherapy is different from natural menopause because it occurs suddenly, unlike normal menopause that gradually occurs over years. The symptoms with chemically induced menopause are more intense because the drugs diminish the hormones made in the ovaries and the adrenal glands. Normal menopause causes a reduction in the ovarian hormones, but not the adrenal glands, which continue to supply some hormones, causing symptoms to be gradual and less severe than those experienced by women who have chemotherapy-induced menopause.

The other important factor to understand about changes in hormonal functioning is the production of testosterone. Testosterone is predominately a male hormone, but females also make testosterone in the ovaries and convert hormones made by the adrenal gland. Testosterone is the hormone that produces sexual desire, controls the ability to experience an orgasm and governs the intensity of the orgasm. When a woman receives treatment with chemotherapy drugs, she has an instant reduction of all female hormones and testosterone from both the ovaries and adrenal glands. Side effects of the reduction of estrogen and progesterone are very apparent—hot flashes, night sweats, mood changes and vaginal dryness. However, the side effect of testosterone reduction, loss of libido, is seldom recognized and is often ignored by the healthcare team. Because the symptoms are experienced by the patient and impact only her and her partner, they are very rarely addressed. By understanding all of these changes, their causes, and learning interventions to reduce side effects, your relationship with your partner should not suffer, but thrive, because of your supportive attitude.

Libido Diminished

After treatment with chemotherapy, a high percentage of women experience a great decrease in libido because of the reduction of testosterone. Sexual thoughts, sexual feelings and sexual day dreams are reduced or are almost non-existent. The ability to experience an orgasm during intercourse is also greatly reduced or absent for most women. Women still experiencing orgasm report that it was reduced in intensity. With the reduction of testosterone, sexual arousal is also a challenge. One woman in the focus group described her sexual desire after chemotherapy as *"that of an 11-year-old girl."* Diminished sexual interest—affecting sexual thoughts, sexual arousal and orgasm—is a common side effect of chemotherapy.

Before chemotherapy treatment, 72 percent of women would experience orgasms, varying from most to all of the time. During treatment, this fell to 21 percent. One year following completion of treatment, this number rose only slightly, to 39 percent, translating into a 54 percent reduction in ability to experience orgasms most or all of the time.

ORGASM ABILITY					
Orgasm	Never	Rarely	Occasionally	Usually	All the Time
Before Treatment	1%	8%	19%	55%	17%
During Treatment	24%	27%	28%	16%	5%
One Year After Treatment	10%	23%	29%	30%	9%

How long does this last? Women who remain in a permanent menopausal state and do not restart their monthly periods after all treatment has ended will continue to struggle with the problem. If a woman has her menstrual periods return, most often a return of libido accompanies them.

It is important to understand that the loss of testosterone—the hormone that causes interest, arousal and orgasm—is the basic problem.

What can be done about these side effects? The testosterone can be brought back into normal range by a trained, experienced healthcare provider who understands the complexity of hormonal balance. Some healthcare providers are unaware of this intervention and contend they don't know if it is safe. However, those women who have had their levels brought back into therapeutic range with testosterone creams report that this brought back the sexual quality of life they enjoyed before treatment. Your partner can ask her healthcare team if they check hormonal levels or supplement testosterone. If not, contact the International Academy of Compounding Pharmacists (1-800-927-4227) and ask for the nearest compounding pharmacy. Your local pharmacy can refer you to the providers in your area who are skilled at testing levels of existing testosterone and prescribe testosterone cream to bring her levels back to normal.

One patient, after years of frustration with her lack of libido, called the International Academy of Compounding Pharmacists and found a local healthcare provider. She received her prescription for the testosterone cream and e-mailed me after two weeks to say that she had not had any results. My advice was to be patient and continue the use. I received an email after five weeks saying, *"My libido is back! This is the best-kept secret in the entire world. Every patient needs to know that there is hope."* After replacement therapy is started, a patient should experience a difference in libido in two to twelve weeks.

Wellbutrin®, an anti-depressant, has also proven helpful in increasing libido and orgasm ability for some women. The medication requires a prescription and is not appropriate for women who experience high levels of anxiety.

Return of libido is a quality of life issue. It has nothing to do with life and death issues, and for this reason it may be ignored. For some couples, return of libido is important to their quality of life. Yet, for others, this is not an issue of high importance. Only the two of you can decide what is best for your relationship. There are no right or wrong answers, only what best meets your needs as a couple. If you find that this is an important issue, keep seeking a healthcare provider who addresses your problems, offers interventions and works to improve your quality of life.

The Orgasm Gap

Males and females have a natural difference in the time between sexual arousal and when orgasm occurs. Understanding this difference is important for a mutually satisfying relationship. Dr. Phil McGraw, Ph.D., states in his book, *Relationship Rescue*:

> *The male's sexual cycle, starting at the contemplation of sex through erection, orgasm and loss of erection, lasts an average of 2.8 minutes. Contrasting this to the female's response curve, which builds more gradually and then plateaus at around seven minutes. Her entire cycle lasts approximately thirteen minutes. The problem is that clitoral dilation and vaginal lubrication usually do not occur until several minutes after the male's cycle is completed. Clearly, you can do the math as well as I can. If the male's cycle lasts 2.8 minutes and the female's cycle lasts 13 minutes, then we have a ten-minute gap in compatibility.*

Average Male & Female Orgasm Cycles

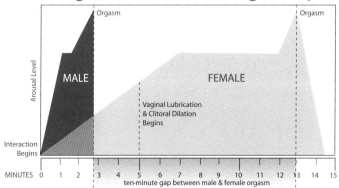

169

You can see from this data, extensive foreplay is needed if a healthy female partner is to experience orgasm. The time needed for female sexual arousal increases even more after chemotherapy. It is essential for a male sexual partner to understand her need and plan for increased foreplay. If increased foreplay is ignored, the sexual encounter can be disappointing and result in painful intercourse for her, causing avoidance of future contact. Wise planning is needed for mutual satisfaction.

When the cause of their reduced libido is explained to patients, they often break into tears, just from having someone recognize and explain the reason for the changes they have endured. As a support partner, recognizing that this is one of the most difficult challenges for women is a great gift of support. The battle they face in the area of sexual functioning is not a choice, but a side effect of treatments.

Vaginal Dryness and Painful Intercourse

Hormonal changes in estrogen reduction cause the vagina to have less lubrication, resulting in vaginal dryness. Estrogen is the hormone that causes the wall of the vagina to be soft and pliable. With the reduction in estrogen, the vagina becomes very dry. Along with the dryness, the vagina will not lubricate adequately during sexual arousal.

VAGINAL DRYNESS
Vaginal dryness from chemotherapy was reported to increase:
▪ 123% during treatment
▪ 134% six months after treatment ended
▪ 160% one year after completion of treatments

If this problem is not understood or corrected, it can result in painful intercourse and possibly a small amount of bleeding after intercourse. Painful intercourse is not pleasant, and bleeding can scare both partners.

PAINFUL INTERCOURSE

Painful intercourse from vaginal dryness increased:

- 126% during treatment

- 137% six months after treatment

- 149% one year after treatment completion

These figures reveal that vaginal dryness with the potential to cause painful intercourse increases after treatment is completed. Therefore, couples should be prepared to deal with the lingering side effects.

There are interventions that can help with dryness and painful intercourse. There are two types of over-the-counter interventions. One is a vaginal moisture-replenishing product (Replens® or Vagisil®) designed to maintain the moisture in the vagina. Vaginal moisturizers are applied inside the vagina on a regular basis, several times a week, to restore and hold moisture. They are like a moisturizer applied to the face to keep moisture in. They are not designed as a lubricant before intercourse.

The other over-the-counter intervention is a vaginal lubricant. Vaginal lubricants are applied prior to intercourse to increase lubrication. Astroglide® is one that is highly recommended by patients as being the most like natural lubrication. Some women are sensitive to lubricants that contain the ingredient glycerin, which causes stinging after application. If this occurs, there are formulas that are glycerin-free. Liquid Silk® is highly recommended by healthcare professionals. It is glycerin-free and also formulated to be bio-static, which means if it is exposed to any bacteria, yeast or fungal spores, it will stop them from spreading. Liquid Silk® can be ordered online. Do not use Vaseline® as a lubricant for intercourse because it can promote vaginal infections.

The female should generously apply the lubricant in the vagina and on the outside on the vaginal lips. As a partner, you can also use the lubricant. Applying the lubricant for your partner can be a sensual part of foreplay. It is important that the lubricant be reapplied as needed during intercourse.

Again, it is very important for a support partner to know that vaginal dryness is not from a patient's lack of desire, but from the inability of her vaginal walls to lubricate properly due to the lack of estrogen. Often, partners may take this reduction of vaginal lubrication as a sign of lack of desire for them as a sexual partner and feel rejected. Some partners feel that the use of a lubricant is a sign that they are not sexually stimulating to their partner. Neither is true. Lack of vaginal lubrication is caused by chemical menopause reducing the estrogen in the body and preventing normal lubrication during the excitement phase of intercourse. This is something the patient cannot control. When support partners express their support and encourage her to use a lubricant for intercourse, this greatly reduces the anxiety of the patient and makes intercourse more comfortable.

Birth Control During Treatment

If your partner is premenopausal, birth control should be discussed with her physician before treatment. Since there is no way to accurately predict if a woman will continue to ovulate and have menstrual periods, birth control is recommended. Chemotherapy drugs could cause birth defects if pregnancy should occur. Birth control pills are not recommended because of their hormonal composition. Spermicidal agents or barrier methods such as condoms or diaphragms are recommended. A decision made by some couples, who have completed their families, is tubal ligation, a minor surgical procedure where a woman's fallopian tubes are cut. This is often done at the time of breast surgery to prevent having to return for a second procedure and additional sedation. Some couples choose that the male partner have a vasectomy.

Tips for Resuming the Sexual Relationship:

- Communicating your continued attraction to her as a sexual partner is the most important foundation for resuming a successful sexual relationship. Find as many ways as possible to convey this message. Say it. Write notes. Send cards. Touch her. Go on special dates together, no matter how simple they may be.

- View the incision area soon after surgery and get this major obstacle to sexual functioning out of the way.

- Verbalize your desire for the resumption of the relationship when she feels ready.

- If surgery is the only treatment, sexual normalcy is solely based on how she views her body image and how she thinks you view her as a sexual partner. Surgery will not impact or cause reduction in the female hormones, causing the multitude of symptoms discussed. The sexual relationship can be resumed as soon as it is mutually desired. Remember to communicate about the potential tenderness of the surgical breast area and what is most comfortable to your partner.

- If radiation therapy follows surgery, an added obstacle may be the fatigue experienced by some women during treatment. This fatigue is not debilitating, but simply a tired feeling that can be helped by additional rest. Some women find that going for treatments daily for weeks is emotionally stressful, and this emotional stress can impact hormonal levels that can affect desire. The best advice is to openly communicate your desire to resume sexual intercourse when she feels ready, but continue to be physically and emotionally close by continuing to touch and hold her.

- For women who have chemotherapy, the challenge is far greater, as we have discussed. You will face additional challenges with addressing hair loss (alopecia), which has proven more difficult for women than dealing with the surgical changes of the breast. Fatigue from chemotherapy may be physically overwhelming during treatments for some women, while others may simply feel tired. Chemotherapy women suffer a double blow to their self-image (surgery and chemotherapy) and need extra assurance that they remain sexually attractive as a partner.

- Plan a time when her energy is at its highest to resume a sexual relationship. The week before her next chemo treatment is a good choice.

- Plan a special time for closeness—a special date, dinner, movie or whatever she enjoys.

- Allow adequate time to touch and stroke her body. Sexual arousal will be slower, and foreplay will need to be longer because of the reduction of female hormones.

- Don't force or ask her to remove her gown or prosthesis if she does not feel comfortable. This may cause her to withdraw emotionally. Some women said that it took several months before they really felt free to participate in intercourse without their scar area covered. Others admitted never wanting to have sexual intercourse without their scar area covered, even though their partner had seen the incision. Removing their clothing resulted in reducing sexual feelings. Do what she feels is comfortable.

■ Prepare for sexual relations by having adequate amounts of a water-based lubricant available. Some women find that when their partners apply the lubricant, it is sexually arousing. Simply ask what she prefers.

■ During treatment with chemotherapy, it is recommended that you use latex condoms.

■ After intercourse, remain close and continue to touch her in a loving way. Assure her that she is still the same loving partner and gives you the same pleasure.

As in all other areas of the breast cancer experience, women and their partners will react differently to each situation. Use these tips as suggestions only. Some partners have said that their sexual relationships were even more gratifying after the cancer experience. Recognizing and understanding the changes following surgery and treatments are a normal part of the recovery process and make you a more sensitive partner. If problems do arise at a later date and you have difficulty working through the changes, trained sexuality counselors are available in most cancer treatment centers or in your community.

Remember...

Surgery and radiation therapy cause only temporary changes in sexual functioning.

Chemotherapy can cause varying levels of effects impacting sexuality, for which you need to understand and prepare to support your partner in finding appropriate interventions.

Resumption of the sexual relationship needs to be approached with sensitivity and planning.

Your understanding of the changes she faces is necessary for the sexual relationship to remain healthy.

"There is no doubt that sexuality, one of the most sensitive and intimate aspects of a relationship, is vulnerable to the ravages of serious illness and its treatment. Many women feel like 'damaged goods' after treatment. Some have lost many external attributes of sexual attractiveness: a breast or hair, the ability to become sexually aroused. They have scars. There are internal losses as well—they feel weak, tired, nauseated and frightened. Added are the possible stresses and strains in the relationship caused by the disease. You may each be losing sleep, worrying in secret so as not to 'trouble' your partner."

—David Spiegel, M.D.

Yes, breast cancer challenges a couple physically, mentally and sexually. However, in the midst of the challenges are the opportunities to share the struggles cancer presents, determined to find resolution by working together. Decide not to become victims of your circumstances. Seek answers by openly communicating with each other and asking questions of your healthcare providers. This is the foundation to turning the challenge into a learning opportunity—an opportunity to grow together and grow closer.

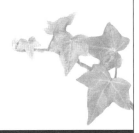

David Spiegel, M.D.

Support Partner Perspectives

"We were newlyweds when Anna was diagnosed; however, that did not mean that the diagnosis did not bring fears about our future as parents. We shared the intense fear that chemotherapy had the potential to rob us of the anticipated joy of having children one day. We still wrestle with the fear that 'if we could have children today, what would happen if Anna had a recurrence?'"

—Brian Cluxton, Support Partner

CHAPTER 19

Future Fertility

*A*t diagnosis, the natural focus is on the patient and getting the most appropriate treatment for her cancer. One of the issues least thought about is the impact of chemotherapy and hormonal therapy cancer treatments on the future fertility of the patient. Most thoughts are focused on the patient and getting the most appropriate treatment for her cancer. However, one of the most important issues for younger women who have not had children, or have not completed their families, is the potential impact on future fertility. It is essential for the patient to ask questions to protect, or plan for, future alternative methods. This chapter will briefly discuss these important issues regarding future fertility.

For women, infertility is the inability to start or maintain a pregnancy. Infertility can occur because of the inability of the ovaries to produce mature eggs (oocytes) for ovulation or from the inability of the body to successfully allow implantation of a fertilized egg into the uterine wall or maintain its growth after implantation.

Women and the Fertility Cycle

When a woman is born, she has all of the eggs she will ever have and will not produce more. When the female hormones gear up at puberty, she experiences the development of secondary sex characteristics, such as pubic hair, breasts and menstruation. Eventually, the menstrual cycles are accompanied by the release of a mature egg at mid-cycle (ovulation); the egg is ready for fertilization by the male sperm. If conception does not occur, or if the fertilized egg does not successfully implant into the uterine wall, the prepared ovarian wall sloughs off, evidenced by the menstrual flow. The entire process begins again for another monthly cycle. Each full cycle averages from 28 – 32 days. Each ovulation reduces the amount of stored eggs. Eventually, the supply of eggs that mature is reduced, ovulation ceases, hormones decrease to pre-menstrual levels and the menstrual periods eventually stop. This cessation of ovarian function, along with the loss of fertility, is called menopause. With menopause come symptoms, not only of infertility, but most often of hot flashes, vaginal dryness, changes in moods, urinary changes and other menopausal symptoms.

Chemotherapy: Potential Impact on Fertility

Surgery has no effect on fertility. It can create stress, which causes temporary changes in the hormonal balance that may temporarily alter ovulation and possibly menstruation. This usually resolves itself in several months. Radiation therapy to the breast has only temporary effects, similar to surgery—stress and fatigue may alter hormonal functioning temporarily, if at all. The major cause of infertility comes from chemotherapy.

Chemotherapy drugs used to treat cancer work by killing rapidly dividing cells throughout the body. Chemotherapy drugs are cytotoxic (cyto=cell, toxic=poison). These drugs kill cancer cells, but in the process also kill healthy, rapidly dividing cells. Shortly after chemotherapy administration, women notice hormonal changes in their bodies. A large majority of women suffer irregular or complete cessation of periods during treatment. Factors that determine the extent of side effects and may also impact future infertility are based on the patient's age, drug type or drug combinations that may compound the effect of toxicity on the body. It is very difficult for an oncologist to accurately predict who will suffer side effects involving their hormonal functioning. For some women, fertility may return after the drugs are discontinued, but for others their infertility may be permanent.

Known Facts to Help in Fertility Prediction

The nearer in age a patient is to menopause, the less likely she is to have hormonal function (menstruation and ovulation) return. The younger the woman, the more likely hormonal function will return.

A class of drugs, called alkylating agents, has a more destructive effect on hormonal function. The most common one used in breast cancer treatment is cyclophosphamide (Cytoxan®). Other drugs that increase infertility in this category are melphalan (Alkeran®) and busulfan (Myleran®). Cisplatin (Platinol®) is usually considered an alkylating agent, even though it works differently than the others in this category, and also impacts fertility.

Addressing Issues of Fertility

Since physicians cannot predict with absolute certainty whose fertility can be permanently affected, there are steps to take to preserve the patient's future ability to have children.

Steps to Help Preserve Fertility:

- The most essential step is discussing with the healthcare team **before** treatments that having children is top priority when making treatment decisions.
- Ask her healthcare team to discuss treatment recommendations and their potential for causing infertility.
- Ask for written information on the subject of chemotherapy and fertility.
- Ask for a referral to a specialist in the area of fertility if she still has questions or concerns.
- Ask for treatment protocols that reduce potential for infertility.
- Explore alternative fertility preservation options.

Fertility Preservation Options:

Embryo Freezing

Hormones (like tamoxifen, safe in breast cancer) are used to stimulate egg production. Mature eggs are removed by a physician in a minor surgical procedure, fertilized in vitro with sperm (in a glass test tube), frozen for future use and then stored. This procedure is called in-vitro fertilization (IVF). Pregnancy rates average 10 to 25 percent with each frozen embryo.

Egg (Oocyte) Freezing

Hormones (like tamoxifen) are used to stimulate egg production. Mature eggs are retrieved by the physician, frozen for future use and then stored without being fertilized. This method is new and at present has an estimated pregnancy success rate of three percent.

Ovarian Retrieval and Transplantation (Research in Progress)

Ovaries are surgically removed by laparoscopy (small incision through the abdomen), divided into small strips, frozen and later transplanted back into the body when fertility is desired. Drugs are given to stimulate ovulation. Some researchers call the process ovarian grafting. This method is experimental but appears to have potential for women who have chemotherapy that will damage their ovaries. Check with your healthcare team on the progress of this research.

Expense and Time Requirements

The procedures for fertility preservation are expensive and usually require several months for egg retrieval, which may delay treatments. At this time, most of the cost is not covered by insurance. During breast cancer decisions, this adds another difficult choice for women who still desire to have a family of their own, but this is an important consideration if future fertility is desired.

It is important to know that some cancers require immediate attention. One of these is inflammatory carcinoma, a cancer that is already advanced because of the involvement of the lymphatic system and requires that treatment start within days of diagnosis. Discuss with her physician if any type of delay would reduce her chances for survival.

Optional Parenthood Choices

Some women find that their main priority during the diagnostic period is the optimal cancer treatment for their cancer and that preserving fertility is not the prominent issue.

Options for Couples Who Wish to Become Parents:

- Use donor eggs if fertility does not return
- Use a surrogate mother
- Adoption

Facts About Pregnancy After Breast Cancer:

- Pregnancy does not seem to reduce patient survival or trigger recurrence.
- Women who have had systemic chemotherapy have been able to conceive and deliver healthy, normal children with the chance of birth defects near that of the normal, untreated population.
- Some physicians suggest that a couple wait six months before attempting pregnancy after regular menstrual periods return. Ask your physician for guidelines.

Questions to Ask Before Chemotherapy:

- What is the predicted impact of the drugs on fertility?

- What percentage of women who take these drugs experience permanent infertility?

- Are there drugs with less potential for infertility that could be used?

- What options does she have to preserve her fertility?

- Do you make referrals to physicians specializing in fertility preservation, if desired?

- If she decides to pursue embryo freezing as an option, will the time required to collect the eggs impact her survival outcomes by delaying treatment for several months?

- If her fertility returns, how long do you suggest she wait before she attempts to become pregnant?

*R*emember...

Future fertility is an issue that might not be discussed by your healthcare team if you do not bring up the subject.

If future fertility is important, ask for information and a referral to a fertility specialist to discuss options best suited to your partner.

Support Partner Perspectives

"Breast cancer was a life-changing event for us. We decided not to brush it under the rug; but instead look for how we could turn it into a positive experience. Today, we both see life completely different than before her diagnosis; we live more in the present. We decided to use our experience working with other young couples diagnosed with cancer through the Young Survival Coalition."

—Brian Cluxton, Support Partner

"My wife had a history of clinical depression, so we had an added area of concern as to how she would handle all of this. She did great in the beginning, but, after chemotherapy, a new kind of tears and withdrawal started. We then tried one-to-one counseling and a breast cancer support group. Talking with, crying with and receiving encouragement from others walking in the same shoes helped her tremendously. ... Breast cancer threatened our relationship. We are taking advantage of our second chance. We've fallen in love all over again. I've seen my wife blossom before my eyes."

—Al Barrineau, Support Partner

CHAPTER 20

Her Emotional Adjustment to Breast Cancer

Breast cancer can serve as a "wake-up call" to life. In one woman's words, *"I realized that I was not going to live forever when I received my diagnosis. I had never stopped to think about it before! But now I live every day to the fullest. No longer will I be a slave to those things in life that were of no consequence."* A new lease on life and a desire to make every day and minute count are often the results of the cancer experience.

One year after her surgery, a patient reminisced, *"Breast cancer was the worst thing that ever happened to me and the best thing that ever happened to me. Even though I hated every change my cancer caused my family to go through, as I reflect, it has brought us a greater degree of happiness and love, and today I would not trade the experience."* Many patients and families report a greater degree of happiness after breast cancer because they decided to concentrate on happiness rather than on things. Facing the dreaded enemy of cancer caused them to refocus their priorities.

This is an opportune time for you to encourage her to look at life and think of things she has always wanted to do, but never did, and make a plan to incorporate them. Encourage her to use breast cancer as the reason to do the things she dreams of and not as an excuse not to. Support her in starting a new hobby, taking a class, getting a pet, planting a flower garden, changing careers, going back to school, becoming a volunteer or planning a trip—whatever she has an interest in doing. A sense of accomplishment will provide a helpful environment for her emotional and physical recovery.

When Emotional Adjustment Becomes Difficult

By the time most women complete their treatments, they have adjusted emotionally to the experience and are putting their lives back into a normal routine. Occasionally, some women have difficulty returning to normal. Even though things are going well physically, and life is returning to a normal routine, emotionally they don't want to move forward and rejoin the family. They seem to be locked into distrust and fear of the future. They don't look forward to the days, months or years ahead. They have lost interest in the things that they once found joyful. Their laughter has been silenced. They find it difficult to plan. They withdraw from family and friends, avoiding social activities when possible. They prefer to spend their time sleeping or in solitude. Some may overeat, while others may have lost their pleasure in food. Some may resort to the overuse of alcohol or drugs to numb their pain. Occasionally, a few may even express that life is not worth living any longer. Somehow, the person you knew before her diagnosis has not yet come back to you emotionally. She has changed greatly.

If you recognize these symptoms in the one you love, you need to alert someone on the healthcare team. Being the person closest to the patient, you will be able to accurately recognize if she is continuing to have problems coping. If this should occur, inform her primary care physician and ask for a referral to a professional counselor.

Depressed people may not even recognize that they are depressed. Even if they do, some patients do not consider their mood disturbances a concern that they should take to the physician. They sometimes think that continuing sad feelings after cancer are normal, but they are not. As a support partner, your close relationship to the patient allows an understanding of what is normal behavior for her and what is not. The first step is understanding how to distinguish normal, reactive depression from clinical depression.

Distinguishing Types of Depression

Normal depression after a loss is an expected reaction. It is described as "feeling blue" or "feeling down" when a person has lost something that is valuable to her physically or emotionally. Breast cancer is certainly a loss to a woman. It is normal for her to cry and feel down at the time of diagnosis and periodically during treatments. During this time, the patient may feel sad but can still enjoy and look forward to parts of her life, such as a family gathering, a movie or seeing a child, grandchild or friend. She still reaches out and shares life's joys and sorrows with those around her. This is a normal, reactive depression—a state of short-term depression that resolves itself.

For some, it is not periodic "feeling blue," but instead an overwhelming constant companion that clouds their view of life. This is clinical depression—an emotional state that does not resolve itself, but remains. Clinical depression is severe depression that causes many physical and emotional changes and needs the intervention of a professional.

Clinical Depression Is Often Manifested By:

- Continual feeling of sadness (after diagnosis, treatments)
- Withdrawing from family and friends socially
- Feeling worthless
- Feeling excessive guilt
- Feeling fearful
- Feeling hopeless about the future
- Being very slow in physical movement or speech
- Feeling constantly jittery or nervous
- Experiencing low energy level; feeling tired all of the time
- Inability to make decisions
- Negative thinking
- Imaginary health problems
- Lacking interest in food or eating excessively
- Disinterest in work or day-to-day activities
- Disinterest in intimacy or sex
- Experiencing insomnia (inability to sleep–wakes early or cannot go to sleep) or sleeps too much
- Having suicidal thoughts (Immediately notify a healthcare professional of suicidal expressions or threats.)

If a person exhibits several (some experts say five or more) of these symptoms for a period of two weeks or longer, her physician should be notified.

Treatment of Clinical Depression

Depression may be treated in several ways. In some cases, counseling may be all that is needed. Counseling identifies weakness in coping skills and works to strengthen them. Often, talking to an understanding person accomplishes much for a depressed person. However, medication may be needed to assist the process. Anti-depressants are often prescribed and will take approximately two weeks to become effective. A class of drugs called SSRIs (Selected Serotonin Reuptake Inhibitors) is very effective for relieving depression. The brand names are Celexa®, Paxil®, Prozac®, Zoloft®, Lexapro® and Luvox®. These drugs not only elevate moods, they have also proven successful in reducing hot flashes, nervousness and decreasing insomnia. Diet and exercise have also been proven to be beneficial in reducing depression and stress. Ask your physician for recommendations.

It is important that the patient understands that depression is **not** a sign of weakness. It is a legitimate condition that is experienced by many people after a major crisis or loss. Most depression is periodic, and short-term counseling and medication will help through this period of adjustment. Identifying and seeking help is the first step to resolving the problem of depression. If you think that this may be occurring, encourage her to call her physician. She may lack the emotional energy to reach out for help. If the depression is severe, you may have to notify her physician.

Events Which Trigger Normal Reactive Depression

After a major loss, there are periods that may be predicted for most cancer patients to experience a return of short-term "feeling blue." As a support partner, it is helpful to be aware of these times and prepare for normal feelings of emotional distress surrounding them.

Post-Treatment Depression

A common time for many patients to experience short-term depression is several weeks after the end of treatment, when they are no longer going to the cancer treatment center on a regular basis. There is no regular monthly contact with the patient's treatment team for the first time since her diagnosis. One patient recalled:

Somehow I felt while I was getting chemotherapy or radiation therapy that they were doing something about my cancer; then all of a sudden I completed my treatments. I thought that this was the time that I had waited for so intensely over the past six months, but to my surprise, I felt frightened. No one was doing anything. I was not seeing anyone. Then the fears overwhelmed me. I didn't know if I could make it on my own. I found myself experiencing many of the sad feelings I had felt at diagnosis; the tears started back. I withdrew emotionally, my appetite left, and I was unable to sleep. But, thankfully, a family member brought my condition to the attention of my physician. I was relieved to know that these feelings happened to many patients at the conclusion of their treatments, and, after talking openly with them, I began to understand.

The conclusion of chemotherapy or radiation therapy treatments is a common time for patients to experience depression. The months of constant contact with the healthcare staff provide a sense of security and socialization for the patient. When treatment ceases and her medical support team is not seen monthly, she becomes very concerned and may feel somewhat alone. Emotionally, this is a very vulnerable time for many patients. It is helpful for you, as a support partner, to plan to spend extra time with the patient or plan a special event at the conclusion of her treatments.

Monitor her emotional state during the weeks and months after treatment. Periods of sadness exhibited by the patient are normal and sometimes last for several consecutive days. If this time turns into weeks, it is advisable to seek assistance for your loved one.

Anniversary Depression
Another common time for short-term depression is around the anniversary date of her diagnosis, surgery or other events involving the cancer diagnosis. These dates may serve as triggers for an "anniversary reaction" and result in a short period of "feeling blue." The date brings back the memories of the event so clearly that the patient finds herself reliving the event to the point that many of the old feelings return. The result may be a brief period of depression.

One psychiatrist, who had bilateral mastectomies, plans a special event for herself on the day of her original diagnosis for breast cancer. She plans a light workday or, if possible, takes the day off and treats herself. She plans for family members or friends to spend this time with her. As a psychiatrist, she knows wise planning can help during these expected times of emotional recall of an event. Yearly regression into many of the old, experienced feelings may happen for years after the event. This is a normal reaction to a traumatic event. Careful planning around these dates to avoid further stress, in addition to your understanding, will help during these times.

Physical Check-Up Depression

Return visits to the physician for check-ups can also renew many of the feelings of depression and anxiety associated with breast cancer. Many women experience high levels of anxiety for several days surrounding their return visits to the physician for check-ups. Know that this reaction is normal. Allow her these brief periods of emotional regression. Check to see if she needs you to be with her for these check-ups. If so, plan to accompany her or arrange to have a friend or family member go with her to the physician. Her greatest fear is that of recurrence. It is most helpful if you both understand and talk about this.

When Treatments End

The breast cancer experience will have changed many things for the patient and those closest to her. Understanding and recognizing some of the major emotional traps of post-treatment depression, anniversary reactions and return physician visits will allow the two of you to plan wisely to maneuver through the brief emotional storms.

By the time surgery, treatments and reconstruction (if chosen) are completed, you both will have been under extended stress. Do not be surprised to find yourself suffering from exhaustion when it is all over. When treatment ends, find out what schedule of tests and visits will monitor her health in the future and mark your calendar. Then try to put breast cancer out of your focus for a while. This is a time to plan something special for the two of you to enjoy together.

Support Partner Perspectives

"Mom's cancer experience changed her. It taught her that caring for herself was also necessary along with caring for everyone else. She had always cared for the family, often neglecting her own needs. She now takes the opportunity to take care of her health and get rest when needed. What it didn't change was her attitude toward life. Her attitude was always 'Don't give up.' Her cancer did impact me. It showed that moms never stop caring for their children, no matter what their circumstances are in life. During the time when she was struggling with the toll chemotherapy had taken on her energy, she never stopped encouraging and caring for my siblings and me. Cancer gave her the opportunity to show us what she really was—a role model for handling life's unexpected challenges."

—Krystle Brown-Shaw, Support Partner

Remember...

Normal (reactive) depression is expected after a major loss.

Support partners should learn to recognize clinical depression, which needs the attention of a healthcare professional.

Anniversary dates, treatment completion and return office visits can cause a reactive depression that may last for several days. Wise planning and support can help reduce the impact.

Plan a special treat after surgery and treatments end. You both deserve it!

Support Partner
Perspectives

"Surgery, chemotherapy and reconstruction were all behind us. Yet there was a cloud of fear over our lives—recurrence. Finding the proper balance between necessary follow-up care and obsession with recurrence can prove a challenge, especially the first few years. The new appreciation for each other and life itself will be lost if you don't control and deal with your fears."

—Al Barrineau, Support Partner

"I consciously choose not to think about recurrence; it is too painful emotionally. Anna monitors her health and follows her doctor's recommendations for follow-up. We choose to enjoy life today and not dwell on a potential disaster that could be lurking in our future. Personally, I don't think of that as denial, but rather as a healthy way to cope with what you cannot control."

—Brian Cluxton, Support Partner

"I know cancer can come back after it's treated. I think about this, and a sense of fear fills my heart. However, Mom also knows this and her attitude is, 'If it comes back, we will have to get it treated again.' I don't ever want to go through this again, but somehow, I find strength in Mom's attitude. If I have to do it, I can. So, I will simply enjoy today and leave that fear in its proper perspective."

—Krystle Brown-Shaw, Support Partner

Managing the Fear of Recurrence

*A*t a time when the battle with treatment for breast cancer is over and life can resume some sense of normalcy, the fear of recurrence can seem like a dark, black cloud. This fear can rob women of their sense of safety and pose a great obstacle for happiness, adding much stress to relationships. This was the most commonly expressed fear by support partners of patients I worked with in support groups, and the number one fear of breast cancer survivors. Fear of recurrence is a shared fear and one that is often not discussed. It is like the "pink elephant" in the room that no one mentions, yet everyone is aware of its presence.

To gain a sense of control over the fear of recurrence, it is helpful if you take steps to manage it. The first step is to acknowledge your fear. The second step is to know that the patient has the same fear. She, too, has to deal with this fear that robs joy from the future. It will be very helpful if you can face this obstacle as a team. Talking together about the need to rationally approach the problem will be the foundation for your plan.

Managing the Fear of Recurrence

How do the two of you manage the fear of recurrence? Denial is certainly not the answer. Recurrence is the most common fear of patients and their support partners. It is a legitimate fear of the future. In fact, when it is not contemplated, there is a danger that you are not dealing with the reality of a breast cancer diagnosis. No one can ever guarantee a patient that there is no more cancer in her future. The greatest problem

I have encountered is the fact that most women, and those who support them, do not have an accurate understanding of the realistic risks of recurrence. Most often, fears are exaggerated to a degree far greater than the truth, causing undue anxiety.

The first step to managing fear is finding accurate information. There are guidelines that can help predict the risk of recurrence. You need to know these risks. To begin finding truth about her risk, talk with her physician. You cannot manage what you don't know. This information must come from her healthcare team and not from the media or well-meaning friends. Accurate information is necessary.

Management Strategies for Fear of Recurrence

Plan to have the discussion with the healthcare team near the end of her treatments, or make an appointment to talk about her particular risks. Some support partners feel a need to talk to the physician in private about the patient's risks. Decide what will best meet your needs.

MAJOR SURVIVOR CHALLENGES

Focus group participants were asked to rank their greatest challenge from a pre-selected list of potential problems. Participants ranked major challenges as follows:

- 56% Fear of recurrence
- 23% Side effects of treatment
- 8% Relationships
- 7% Insurance
- 4% Job loss
- 2% Social or career barriers

As indicated in the chart above, the fear of recurrence was overwhelmingly the number one challenge of women in the focus groups. Most women and their support partners will find that it is usually one of the main challenges they face after treatment completion.

Recurrence Questions:

- **What are her risks for recurrence?**
  Most often, people overestimate the risk when there is not a frank discussion with the healthcare team. You need to know the truth. Remember to use statistical data as a guideline, not as an absolute fact. Every woman is an individual and does not necessarily fit the statistical tables.

- **How often will she return to you for a check-up?**
  Return visits for check-ups vary. They are usually every three months after treatment and are gradually reduced, if no problems arise.

- **What diagnostic tests do you plan to perform during these check-ups?**
  On return physician visits, a careful history of events since the last visit and a physical exam are performed. Physicians have various schedules of when to perform blood work studies, mammograms, bone scans, liver scans, CT scans, chest X-rays, etc. Ask what scheduled tests are planned as follow-up care. Women are often frightened when they are scheduled for some diagnostic tests. They think the physician is suspicious of a recurrence, when in reality the test is a regularly scheduled, follow-up test for all patients.

- **What signs and symptoms do we need to report?**
  Your physician will tell you the most likely signs of recurrence, according to the type of breast cancer the patient had. Cancers vary in their likelihood of recurring in a specific manner. Your physician can help you know which symptoms need immediate medical attention.

- **What can we do to maximize her recovery?**
  Ask about diet, exercise, breast self-exam and medications she should or should not take (example: estrogen-type medications). Physicians will often recommend professionals to work with the patient to learn about diet, exercise programs and breast self-exam. Encourage the patient to participate in learning, but do not force her. Patients often need a time for emotional retreat and find it stressful to take on any new challenges immediately after treatment is completed.

One of the ways you may help is to offer to participate in some of these recovery strategies. You may both wish to change your dietary habits or start an exercise program together.

Breast Cancer Recurrence

The majority of breast cancer recurrences occur within the first five years, with an estimate of 60 to 80 percent occurring in the first three years after treatment. Therefore, it is very important that the patient keeps her appointments with her physician for close monitoring of her health. Recurrence is highly unpredictable—no one can say absolutely if and when. Her physicians have given the best protection against recurrence through recommended treatments. The next step is a partnership for monitoring her future health for any signs of recurrence.

Breast Cancer Recurrence Types

If breast cancer recurs, her cancer will be re-staged. There are three types of recurrence:

- **Local recurrence** is cancer that returns to the local area of removal. This type of recurrence is considered failure of primary treatment and not a sign of a more aggressive cancer. This happens because it is impossible to destroy every cancer cell during surgery and radiation. A local recurrence does not change the stage of her cancer.

- **Regional recurrence** is when cancer spreads outside the breast and underarm lymph nodes. This spread may be to the chest muscles, internal mammary nodes underneath the breastbone or in the nodes above the collarbone.

- **Distant recurrence** is when the cancer is found in a distant site such as the bones, lungs, liver, brain or other sites in the body.

Monitoring Her Future Health

The American Society of Clinical Oncology (ASCO) recommends follow-up guidelines for the management of a breast cancer patient and a follow-up schedule for physician visits.

Recommended Surveillance Guidelines:

- Physician physical examination, including complete patient history
- Patient education about signs and symptoms to report on a scheduled basis
- Breast self-exam and mammography
- Pelvic examination
- Diagnostic/surveillance testing when a patient has symptoms that indicate a need

Recommended Physician Visit Schedule:

- 1 – 3 years past treatment, every 3 – 6 months
- 4 – 5 years past treatment, every 6 – 12 months
- 6 years or more past treatment, every 12 months

Returning to the physician for a physical exam and update of the patient's history is the most important way to monitor for recurrence. It has been proven that a physician's exam and review of recent physical changes reported by the patient is the number one way that most recurrences are detected. The patient can make the most of her appointment by preparing to report any changes experienced since her last visit. It is helpful if she keeps a record of any changes so she doesn't forget. These changes should be reported early in the visit so that the physician will have the time to further evaluate the change.

During the exam, her doctor will look for any physical changes that relate to her general health and/or any symptoms that may suggest cancer has recurred locally or spread to another part of her body (systemic disease). In addition to performing a careful breast exam, the doctor will closely examine the patient's entire chest wall and check for lymph node enlargement in other areas of her body. Her heart and lungs will be listened to, and her abdomen, liver, spleen, neck and other areas will be checked for swelling or tenderness. The doctor will also check for any changes in her neurological (nerve) functioning that may be associated with recurrence.

Signs and Symptoms to Report for Potential Local Recurrence:

- Change in size, shape or contour of the lumpectomy breast
- Nipple discharge that is clear or bloody
- Nipple inversion
- New onset of breast pain
- A new lump that may feel like a small pea in the breast or mastectomy scar area
- Thickening in breast tissues or on chest wall after mastectomy
- Changes in the skin: dimpling (pulling in of skin), scaly appearance, rash, redness or any discoloration on breast or chest wall
- A lump or thickening in the underarm area

Monitoring for Potential Regional or Distant Recurrence:

- New lump or thickening in area above the collarbone
- Chronic bone pain or tenderness in an area
- Chest pain with shortness of breath
- Chronic cough
- Persistent abdominal pain or abdominal swelling
- Headaches, dizziness, fainting or rapid changes in vision
- Increasing fatigue unrelated to treatments
- Inability to control urine or bowels
- Persistent nausea or loss of appetite
- Changes in weight, especially weight loss

Encourage the patient to report any other changes that she observes. The most common way recurrence is discovered is when a patient reports symptoms or changes she has experienced in her health. Don't ignore any change as being unimportant. Instead, let the physician or nurse make that decision. What may seem unimportant may be important to the healthcare team.

Additional diagnostic tests will be recommended after the physician's assessment and physical exam if the tests would be helpful to further explore or clarify any changes. With this open partnership, any recurrence should be detected early.

Potential Diagnostic Tests

The physician may supplement the patient's physical exam with additional diagnostic tests if any reported symptoms warrant the need for more diagnostic information. Diagnostic tests may include MRI or dedicated breast MRI, PET scan, computed tomography (CAT scan), chest X-rays, bone scans, liver ultrasound or tests for breast cancer tumor markers such as CA 15-3, CA27.29 or CEA.

Communicating Fears to Healthcare Team

Most physicians have a nurse who is qualified to answer many questions by patients and to refer those that need a physician's attention. Identify this person. It is normal during the first few years to think that every pain is a sign of recurrence. Managing these fears is best accomplished by communicating with the person who can appropriately evaluate your concerns. Utilize this fear management technique. If you have any questions, call and ask this person immediately, rather than worrying and waiting until the next appointment date. Use your healthcare team as your advisor as to whether there is a cause for concern when symptoms arise.

Communicating About Recurrence Fears

After getting accurate information from your healthcare team, the next step will be the need to build an open, honest relationship about these concerns. The patient needs to feel that she can share her physical concerns and fears without "upsetting" you. Women often feel uncomfortable sharing physical symptoms; they don't want to worry anyone. However, you can help monitor her health if she feels free to tell you how she is feeling or if she has any physical changes occurring.

As mentioned previously, she also needs to have the freedom to verbalize her fears in times in which she is vulnerable—check-ups, anniversary dates and times of depression. Her road to recovery may have some detours through anxiety and days of depression. This is normal. You can help by recognizing these times, allowing her to talk and giving her support.

Help her plan a stress-free schedule, if possible, around anniversary dates and checkups. She will vividly remember these times. Your acknowledgment by being supportive will be very helpful to her emotional recovery. Plan a special treat—a meal out, a single flower, a note telling her of your love—to make these times easier. Remember, she is not looking to you for miracles, only for your understanding and support.

Managing Your Anxieties

We have been discussing managing fears of recurrence and how you can help the patient by allowing open communication. Yet, a very vital part of your personal fear management is finding someone with whom you can openly share your fears and feelings. You will find this type of person in support groups, friends, professional counselors and spiritual counselors. Look for these sources of support among those who truly understand, and take full advantage of the help they offer. One support partner said:

> *We need to understand the needs of the ones we love, but we also need to understand and meet our own needs for support. I found this source in a support group of other support partners. That is when I finally managed to get my fears under control. … I needed support, too.*

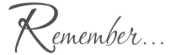emember...

The fear of recurrence is a joy robber. Both of you must address it with accurate information and open communication for optimal emotional recovery.

Accurate information is obtained by consulting with the healthcare team concerning risks and signs and symptoms that need to be reported.

She will have predictable times when her fears of recurrence increase—physical check-ups and anniversary dates of diagnosis or surgery/treatment. Wise planning can reduce the intensity of her fear.

She is not looking to you for miracles, only loving support.

Facing Fear

"To fight fear, ACT. To increase fear—wait, put off, postpone."

—**David Joseph Schwartz**

"Fear is conquered by action. When we challenge our fears, we defeat them. When we grapple with our difficulties, they lose their hold upon us. When we dare to face the things which scare us, we open the door to freedom."

—**Wynn Adams**

"You gain strength, courage and confidence by every experience in which you really stop to look fear in the face. The danger lies in refusing to face the fear, in not daring to come to grips with it. You must do something you think you cannot do."

—**Eleanor Roosevelt**

"Fear can keep us up all night, but faith makes one fine pillow."

—**Philip Gulley**

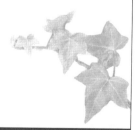

Support Partner
Perspectives

"Mom's breast cancer was an unwanted event that came into our family's life. It was unexpected, and we were unprepared. We learned to deal with it day by day. Some days were good—some days were not so good. In the midst of the experience, we grew even closer emotionally. The roles changed as I, the child, supported and cared for the mother. We saw life from a new and different perspective—the child as the caregiver. This new perspective confirmed that no matter what we faced, we could make it if we drew our strength from each other. We learned that today we may be the strong one and tomorrow we may be the needy one, in need of support. We also learned that this is the strength found in families. We will be there whenever we are needed; bringing our love, willingly, to support the one we love."

—Krystle Brown-Shaw, Support Partner

"For us, the whole breast cancer experience has almost been a blessing; I know that is hard for you to believe or even think it's possible right after the diagnosis of the one you love. It takes time, but today we have a closer relationship than ever before. We have learned a lot about our relationship, and I learned a lot about myself that I would not have learned without the experience."

—Brian Cluxton, Support Partner

CHAPTER 22

Shared Insights on Coping

*W*orking as a Breast Health Navigator, I have had the opportunity to observe hundreds of support partners as they worked through the breast cancer experience with the ones they loved. It is not an easy task. Being a support partner is one of the most difficult tasks because there is no training. There are very few guidelines to allow you to evaluate if you are doing the right things to truly support her. It is on-the-job training that requires a delicate balance of caring for someone else while also caring for yourself.

I have observed that some support partners become so hyper-attentive in their new role of endeavoring to meet all of the patient's physical and emotional needs that they forget to take care of their own. There are some who feel too inadequate to even attempt to fill the role and fail to even try to make things better. They fall into a pattern of denial or avoidance and leave the patient to depend on someone else for support through the crisis. The majority, however, muster all of the emotional muscle available and learn to become the support partner the patient needs.

Through my work, I have seen wonderful things happen to relationships. I have seen relationships grow into a deeper commitment. I have witnessed a new level of love and trust develop between the patient and the support partner. One patient shared about her spouse, *"We feel like we did when we were dating 25 years ago. We can't wait to see each other at the close of the day. Somehow we had gotten so busy we had lost each other in a flurry of careers and activities. Breast cancer gave us back the gift of our love for each other."* Many relationships experience this renewal. Adult children, siblings and friends who served as support partners have also expressed that the experience, even though challenging at times, proved to draw them closer emotionally.

"It took our relationship to a new level of love and appreciation for each other," a daughter shared about her mom.

Working closely with support partners, I have had the privilege of listening as they have shared things that made a difference in helping them in their new role. I asked some of them to share their best advice in an effort to make your journey a little easier.

Advice From Other Support Partners

- Acknowledge the patient's emotions, as well as your own. Don't stifle them. Don't try to be too positive; this can be as difficult for her as it would be if you were depressed.

- Find someone you can trust—someone who understands your needs— and talk with that person. We all need support; it makes life easier to bear.

- Gather up-to-date information on the disease, and become knowledgeable of the basic decisions that need to be made. Often women are paralyzed with fear and cannot take these steps. Knowledge increases your sense of control and allows you to become partners with the healthcare team.

- Recruit needed help from family and friends. They want to be helpful. They appreciate it when you tell them, specifically, what your needs are at the time. Don't make them guess. Be precise. They appreciate knowing exactly what they can do to reduce the burden and be helpful.

- Stay organized with your record-keeping. Get a calendar and keep accurate records. This will help when insurance companies and hospitals are billing you for services—often months later.

- Rearrange your previous priorities, realizing it will be for a limited period of time, not forever. A golf game may need to be exchanged for a walk together or an outing to the mall for her emotional support. You may even need to take an occasional "mental health" day from work to take care of your own emotional and physical needs.

- Plan special and fun times for the two of you. Often, recreation and fun times are abandoned during treatment, but this should not be the case. Be creative in how recreation needs change because of limited amounts of energy, but plan some time of diversion for the two of you. During chemotherapy treatments, the best time is several days before her next treatment.

- Seek feedback. There is a careful balance between communication and silence, withdrawal and over-involvement, separateness and togetherness, attentiveness and emotional distance. People have different involvement needs. Be sure that you are not expending too much energy in areas that she may feel are unnecessary.

- Take care of your physical health. As your focus changes to meet her needs during surgery and treatment, be sure that you remember to watch your diet and eat regular, balanced meals; avoid overeating or skipping meals; get an adequate amount of sleep; avoid alcohol, smoking or drug use (these will lower your physical resistance); and maintain some type of exercise. Exercise is one of the best ways to reduce stress. Take walks, ride bikes with the children or go to the gym. This can relieve a great deal of tension.

- Add the magic. Say, *"I love you,"* often, and be as creative as possible in conveying the message.

- One couple shared, *"Breast cancer gave us the opportunity to fall in love all over again."* Use this time as an opportunity to rekindle your relationship.

- One support partner expressed, *"Today, I am a different person. I know what pain of the heart feels like, and, from knowing pain personally, I have grown into a stronger, more sensitive and compassionate person—a person I like better."*

Indeed, breast cancer is an unexpected journey that is filled with many challenges for you and the one you love. Yet, as you journey together, you will find that the lessons learned are invaluable. Without a doubt, you would never volunteer to undergo the experience again. However, emerging from the journey, you will both find that you have changed. Cancer is a defining and refining experience; one that allows you to view life from a different perspective. This new perspective adds much richness to everyday life.

As you serve in the supporting role, remember, that your support serves as the place where she is protected from the emotional storms and because of this, she manages to flourish in spite of the challenges endured.

My blessings on your journey together,

Judy

Support Partner Perspectives

"*Finding the proper balance in your life is a challenge, especially in the first few years after diagnosis. The new appreciation for each other and life itself will be lost if you don't control your own fears. Take interest in her emotional, as well as physical, recovery, but do the same for yourself. You aren't going to be much help to her if you don't take care of yourself. … At diagnosis I thought we were given a death sentence. Today, I know that doesn't have to be the case. With the right medical team, educating yourself about cancer, and faith, there can be a better quality of life after breast cancer. Harriett now serves as a Reach To Recovery Volunteer, visiting, educating and encouraging newly diagnosed patients as they begin their new battle with breast cancer. I gladly share my experiences with new support partners. We don't take each other for granted anymore. We now have a regular habit of dating—another good thing that came out of the experience. Our relationship has priority.*"

—Al Barrineau, Support Partner

Resources

American Cancer Society (ACS)
1-800-ACS-2345 (1-800-227-2345)
www.cancer.org
Provides free, written information on breast cancer, support group information and referrals to Reach to Recovery program for peer interaction.

Caring Bridge
www.caringbridge.org
Non-profit Web service that provides a free Web site to anyone going through a health crisis, treatment or recovery.

National Cancer Institute (NCI)
www.cancer.gov
The National Cancer Institute maintains a cancer treatment database, providing prognostic, stage and treatment information on more than 1,000 protocol (treatment) summaries.

National Comprehensive Cancer Network:
Breast Cancer Treatment Guidelines for Patients
www.nccn.org
Decision trees included on this site aid patients in choosing treatment and follow-up options. Also available in Spanish.

Susan G. Komen for the Cure
1-877-GO-KOMEN (1-877-465-6636)
www.komen.org
Offers information on all areas of breast cancer treatment and support.

The Young Survival Coalition (Young Women)
1-877-972-1011
www.youngsurvival.org
An advocacy and awareness organization for young women who are diagnosed with breast cancer. The group offers support, information and education.

Recommended Reading

The Human Side of Cancer: Living With Hope, Coping With Uncertainty
Jimmie C. Holland, M.D.; Sheldon Lewis
Publisher: Harper Paperbacks; 10/2001
ISBN: 006093042X (Available on Amazon)

Living Beyond Limits
David Spiegel, M.D.
Publisher: Random House; 1994
ISBN: 9780449909409 (Available on Amazon)

The Portable Therapist: Wise and Inspiring Answers to the Questions People in Therapy Ask the Most...
Susanna McMahon, Ph.D.
Publisher: Dell; 07/1994
ISBN: 0440506034 (Available on Amazon)

Relationship Rescue: A Seven-Step Strategy for Reconnecting With Your Partner
Phillip C. McGraw, Ph.D.
Publisher: Hyperion Books; 2000
ISBN: 0786866314 (Available on Amazon)

Sexuality and Fertility After Cancer
Leslie R. Schover, Ph.D.
Publisher: Wiley; 09/1997
ISBN: 0471181943 (Available on Amazon)

Timeless Healing
Herbert Benson, M.D.; Marg Stark
Publisher: Scribner; 03/1997
ISBN: 0684831465 (Available on Amazon)

RECOMMENDED READING

CHILDREN

Heaven's Not a Crying Place: Teaching Your Child About Funerals, Death, and the Life Beyond
Joey O'Connor
Publisher: Baker Books
ISBN: 0800756436 (Available on Amazon)

Talking With Kids About Cancer
Dave Dravecky
Publisher: Outreach of Hope
(Available at www.OutreachofHope.org)

PATIENTS

Breast Cancer Treatment Handbook, Seventh Edition
Judy C. Kneece, RN, OCN
Publisher: EduCare Publishing Inc.; 2009
ISBN: 9781886665231
(Available at www.educareinc.com)

Cancer: 50 Essential Things to Do, Third Edition
Greg Anderson
Publisher: Plume; 02/2009
ISBN: 0452290104 (Available on Amazon)

Chicken Soup for the Breast Cancer Survivor's Soul: Stories to Inspire, Support and Heal
Jack Canfield, Mark Victor Hansen, Mary Olsen Kelly
Publisher: Health Communications; 10/2006
ISBN: 0757305210 (Available on Amazon)

The Triumphant Patient: Become an Exceptional Patient in the Face of Life-Threatening Illness
Greg Anderson
Publisher: iUniverse, Inc.; 10/2000
ISBN: 0595131050 (Available on Amazon)

Glossary

It is important to understand the medical terminology related to diagnosis and treatments. The following is a list of the most common medical terms used in breast cancer. If you do not understand the technical language used by the healthcare team, ask them to explain what they mean. Understanding the terms will enable you to make intelligent decisions.

ABSOLUTE RISK REDUCTION — Absolute number of patients who will benefit from a treatment.

ADENOCARCINOMA — A form of cancer that involves cells from the lining of the walls of many different organs of the body. Breast cancer is a type of adenocarcinoma.

ADJUVANT TREATMENT — Treatment that is added to increase the effectiveness of a primary treatment. In cancer, adjuvant treatment usually refers to chemotherapy, hormonal therapy or radiation therapy after surgery to increase the likelihood of killing all cancer cells.

ALKYLATING AGENT — Type of chemotherapy drug used in cancer treatment.

ALOPECIA — Refers to hair loss as a result of chemotherapy or from radiation therapy administered to the head. Hair loss from chemotherapy is temporary. Hair loss from radiation may be permanent.

ALTERNATIVE MEDICINE — Treatments used instead of standard treatments. They generally are not recognized by the medical community as standard or conventional medical approaches.

ANALGESIC — Medicine given to control pain; for example: Aspirin or Tylenol®.

ANEMIA — Condition marked by a decrease in the blood component hemoglobin that causes symptoms of fatigue, weakness, dizziness, inability to concentrate and shortness of breath. Many chemotherapy drugs cause a reduction in hemoglobin levels.

ANESTHESIA — Medication that causes entire or partial loss of feeling or sensation.

ANESTHESIOLOGIST — A doctor who specializes in giving drugs to prevent or relieve pain during surgery or other procedures being done in the hospital.

ANDROGEN — A male sex hormone. Androgens may be used in patients with breast cancer to treat recurrence of the disease.

ANEUPLOID — The characteristic of having either fewer or more than the normal number of chromosomes in a cell. This is an abnormal cell.

ANOREXIA — Severe, uncontrolled loss of appetite.

ANTIEMETIC — A medicine that prevents or relieves nausea and vomiting; used during, and sometimes after, chemotherapy.

ANTIMETABOLITES — Anticancer drugs that interfere with the process of DNA production, thus preventing cell division.

ASYMPTOMATIC — Without obvious signs or symptoms of disease. While cancer may cause symptoms and warning signs, it may develop and grow without producing any symptoms, especially in its early stages.

ATYPICAL CELLS — Not usual; abnormal. Cancer is the result of atypical cell division.

AUTOLOGOUS — Tissue from your own body.

AXILLA — The armpit.

AXILLARY DISSECTION — Surgical removal of lymph nodes from the armpit. The tissue removed is sent to the pathologist to determine if the breast cancer has spread outside of the breast. The number of nodes dissected varies during surgery. Your physician can tell you how many nodes were removed.

AXILLARY NODES — Lymph nodes in the axilla (underarm). These nodes may be cut out and examined during surgery to see if the cancer has spread past the breast. The number of nodes in this area varies.

AXILLARY SAMPLING — Procedure where lymph nodes are removed from under the arm during breast cancer surgery to evaluate if cancer is present.

BENIGN TUMOR — An abnormal growth that is not cancerous and does not spread to other parts of the body.

BILATERAL — Pertains to both sides of the body. For example, bilateral breast cancer would be on both sides of the body or in two breasts.

BIOLOGICAL RESPONSE MODIFIER — Treatment used that alters the body's natural response to stimulate bone marrow to make specific blood cells. Referred to as a colony stimulating factor.

BIOPSY — The surgical removal of a small piece of tissue or a small tumor for microscopic examination to determine if cancer cells are present. A biopsy is the most important procedure in diagnosing cancer.

BIOTHERAPY — Treatments used to stimulate the body's immune system.

BLOOD COUNT — A test to measure the number of red blood cells (RBCs), white blood cells (WBCs) and platelets in a blood sample.

BONE SCAN — A procedure in which a trace amount of radioactive substance is injected into the bloodstream to illuminate the bones under a special camera to see if the cancer has spread to the bones.

BRCA 1 AND BRCA 2 — Genes identified to increase risk of hereditary breast cancer.

BREAST CANCER — A potentially fatal tumor, because of its ability to leave the breast, go to other vital organs and continue to grow, if it is not removed from the body. These are breast cells that are abnormal with uncontrolled growth.

BREAST IMPLANT — A round or teardrop-shaped sac inserted into the body to restore the shape of the breast. May be filled with saline water or synthetic material.

BREAST-CONSERVING SURGERY — Surgery that removes cancer while saving the basic cosmetic appearance of the breast, including the nipple and areola.

CAM — Stands for Complementary, Alternative Medicine.

CANCER — A general term used to describe more than 100 different uncontrolled growths of abnormal cells in the body. Cancer cells have the ability to continue to grow, invade and destroy surrounding tissue, leave the original site and travel via lymph or blood systems to other parts of the body, where they can set up new cancerous tumors.

CANCER CELL — A cell that divides and reproduces abnormally with uncontrolled growth. This cell can break away and travel to other parts of the body and set up another site; this is referred to as metastasis.

CAPSULAR CONTRACTURE — Fibrous tissues that form around an implant and cause changes in the shape of the implant and may cause pain.

CARCINOEMBRYONIC ANTIGEN (CEA) — A blood test used to monitor women with metastatic breast cancer to help determine if the treatment is working. This is not a test specific for cancer.

CARCINOGEN — Any substance that initiates or promotes the development of cancer. For example, asbestos is a proven carcinogen.

CARCINOMA — A form of cancer that develops in tissues covering or lining organs of the body, such as the skin, the uterus, the lung or the breast.

CARCINOMA IN SITU — An early stage of development, when the cancer is still confined to the tissues of origin and has not spread outside the area. In situ carcinomas are highly curable.

CAT SCAN OR CT SCAN — An imaging exam that uses X-rays to create cross-sectional pictures of the body.

CELL — The basic structural unit of all life. All living matter is composed of cells.

CHEMOTHERAPY — Treatment of cancer by use of chemicals. Usually refers to drugs used to treat cancer.

CLINICAL TRIAL — A scientific study, generally involving a large number of test subjects (or patients), that is conducted to prove or determine the effectiveness of a drug or treatment program. Limited experimental evidence and preliminary studies prior to the clinical trial have shown or suggested the potential effectiveness and usefulness of the drug or treatment.

COBRA — Consolidated Omnibus Budget Reconciliation Act of 1985. A health insurance available if you are terminated or laid off from your job. This health insurance would remain in effect for a period of 18 months after the job is terminated.

COMBINATION CHEMOTHERAPY — Treatment consisting of the use of two or more chemicals to achieve maximum kill of tumor cells.

COMBINED MODALITY THERAPY — Two or more types of treatments used to supplement each other. For instance, surgery, radiation, chemotherapy, hormonal therapy or immunotherapy may be used separately or together for maximum effectiveness.

COMPLEMENTARY MEDICINE — Treatment often used to enhance or complement standard treatments. For example, massage therapy.

COMPLETE BLOOD COUNT (CBC) — A laboratory test to determine the number of red blood cells, white blood cells, platelets, hemoglobin and other components of a blood sample.

COMPUTERIZED TOMOGRAPHY SCANS — Commonly called CT or CAT scans. These specialized X-ray studies detect cancer or metastasis.

CONTRAST AGENT — Compounds used to improve the visibility of internal bodily structures during an X-ray image or an MRI.

CYTOLOGY — The study of cells that have been sloughed off, cut out or scraped off of organs; cells are microscopically examined for signs of cancer.

CYTOTOXIC — Drugs that can cause the death of cancer cells. Usually refers to drugs used in chemotherapy treatments.

DELAYED RECONSTRUCTION — Reconstruction performed at any time after breast cancer surgery.

DEPRESSION — A mental condition marked by ongoing feelings of sadness, despair, loss of energy, difficulty dealing with normal daily life, feelings of worthlessness and hopelessness, loss of pleasure in activities, changes in eating or sleeping habits, and thoughts of death or suicide.

DETECTION — The discovery of an abnormality in an asymptomatic or symptomatic person.

DEXA SCAN — Dual Energy X-ray Absorptiometric scan. An imaging test that measures bone density to diagnose osteoporosis.

DIAGNOSIS — The process of identifying a disease by its characteristic signs, symptoms and laboratory findings. With cancer, the earlier the diagnosis is made, the better the chance for a cure.

DIEP RECONSTRUCTION — A type of breast reconstruction in which blood vessels called Deep Inferior Epigastric Perforators (DIEP) are removed, along with the skin and fat connected to them, from the lower abdomen. Muscle is not used.

DIFFERENTIATED — The similarity between a normal cell and the cancer cell; defines what degree of change has occurred. Cancer cells that are well differentiated are close to the original cell and are usually less aggressive. Poorly differentiated cells have changed more and are more aggressive.

DIPLOID — The characteristic of having two sets of chromosomes in a cell. This is normal for a breast cell.

DNA — One of two nucleic acids (the other is RNA) found in the nucleus of all cells. DNA contains genetic information on cell growth, division and cell function.

DOSE-DENSE CHEMOTHERAPY — Same amount (dose) of chemotherapy drugs given in a shorter period of time. Usually every two weeks rather than every three weeks.

DOUBLING TIME — The time required for a cell to double in number. Breast cancer has been shown to double in size every 23 to 209 days. It would take one cell, doubling every 100 days, eight to ten years to reach one centimeter (⅜ inch, or the size of the tip of your small finger).

DUCTAL CARCINOMA IN SITU — A cancer inside the ducts of the breast that has not grown through the wall of the duct into the surrounding tissues. Sometimes referred to as a precancer. Good prognosis is involved with in situ cancers.

ENDOCRINE MANIPULATION — Treating breast cancer by changing the hormonal balance of the body to prevent hormone-dependent cancer cells from multiplying.

ESTROGEN — A female hormone, secreted by the ovaries, that is essential for menstruation, reproduction and the development of secondary sex characteristics, such as breasts. Some patients with breast cancer are given drugs to suppress the production of estrogen in their bodies.

ESTROGEN RECEPTOR ASSAY (ERA) — A test that is done on cancerous tissue to see if a breast cancer is hormone-dependent and may be treated with hormonal therapy. The test will reveal if your cancer is estrogen receptor positive or negative.

ESTROGEN RECEPTORS (ER) — Describes cells that have a protein to which the hormone estrogen will bind. Cancer cells that are estrogen receptor positive need estrogen to grow. Tumor is tested by the pathologist after surgery to determine if cells are estrogen positive or estrogen negative.

EXTERNAL BEAM RADIATION — High dose of X-ray beams delivered to the site of cancer by a machine called a linear accelerator.

FAMILIAL CANCER — Cancer occurring in families more frequently than would be expected by chance.

FAMILY AND MEDICAL LEAVE ACT (FMLA) — Law that allows eligible employees to take up to 12 work weeks in any 12-month period off from work for personal illness.

FATIGUE — A condition marked by extreme tiredness and inability to function due to lack of energy.

FERTILITY — The ability to have children.

FLAP NECROSIS — Cell death of flap tissues transplanted from another area of the body during reconstruction; caused by lack of blood supply to the tissues.

FLOW CYTOMETRY — A test done on cancerous tissues that shows the aggressiveness of the tumor. It shows how many cells are in the dividing stage at one time, commonly referred to as the "S" phase, and the DNA content of the cancer, referred to as the ploidy. This reveals how rapidly the tumor is growing.

FREE FLAP — Tissues (skin and fat, with or without muscle) removed from an area of the body that are cut free from their original blood supply and reattached at the new reconstruction site.

FROZEN SECTION — A technique in which a part of the biopsy tissue is frozen immediately, and a thin slice of frozen tissue is mounted on a microscope slide for a diagnostic examination by a pathologist.

FROZEN SHOULDER — Surgical shoulder which has a severely restricted range of motion and is painful.

GAMMA-DETECTION PROBE — Instrument used during sentinel node biopsy to identify radiation uptake of first nodes that drain a tumor.

GENES — Segments of DNA that contain hereditary information that is transferred from cell to cell; genes are located in the nucleus of the cell.

GENETIC — Refers to the inherited pattern located in genes for certain characteristics.

GLUTEUS (GLUTEAL) FLAP — Tissues composed of muscle, fat and blood vessels removed from the buttocks and used to reconstruct the breast.

HEALTHCARE DIRECTIVES — A written document that instructs others about your healthcare wishes, including appointing a healthcare agent and specific healthcare instructions, should you be unable to make decisions on your own.

HEMATOMA — A collection of blood that can form in a wound after surgery, an aspiration or an injury.

HEMOGLOBIN — A component inside red blood cells that binds to oxygen in the lungs and carries it to all of the tissues in the body.

HER2/NEU — <u>H</u>uman <u>e</u>pidermal growth factor <u>r</u>eceptor 2 is a protein identified in breast cancer indicating increased aggressiveness.

HORMONAL THERAPY — Treatment of cancer by alteration of the hormonal balance. Some cancers will only grow in the presence of certain hormones.

HORMONES — Chemicals secreted by various organs in the body that help regulate growth, metabolism and reproduction. Some hormones are used as treatment following surgery for breast, ovarian and prostate cancers.

HORMONE RECEPTOR ASSAY — A diagnostic test to determine whether a breast cancer's growth is influenced by hormones or if it can be treated with hormones.

HOT FLASHES — A sensation of heat and flushing that occurs suddenly. May be associated with menopause or some chemotherapy medications.

IMMEDIATE RECONSTRUCTION — Breast reconstruction performed immediately after breast cancer surgery.

IMMUNE SYSTEM — A complex system by which the body protects itself from outside invaders that are harmful to the body.

IMMUNOLOGY — The study of the body's mechanisms of resistance against disease and invasion by foreign substances—the body's ability to fight a disease.

IMMUNOTHERAPY — A treatment that stimulates the body's own defense mechanisms to combat diseases such as cancer.

IMMUNOSUPPRESSED — Condition of having a lowered resistance to disease. May be a temporary result of lowered white blood cells from chemotherapy administration.

INFILTRATING CANCER — Cancer that has grown through the cell wall of the breast area in which it originated, and into the surrounding tissues.

INFILTRATING DUCTAL CARCINOMA — A cancer that begins in the mammary duct and has spread to areas outside of the duct.

INFLAMMATORY CARCINOMA — Very aggressive cancer in the lymphatics of the breast; requires immediate treatment with chemotherapy for disease control.

INFORMED CONSENT — Process of explaining to the patient the risks and complications of a procedure or treatment before it is done. Most informed consents are written and signed by the patient or a legal representative.

IN SITU — In place, localized and confined to one area. A very early stage of cancer.

INTEGRATIVE MEDICINE — Combination of both evidence-based or mainstream medicine and complementary therapies such as massage, yoga, etc.

INTERNAL BREAST RADIATION — Radiation therapy that places the radiation source inside of the breast for short periods of time; given after breast cancer surgery.

INTERNAL MAMMARY NODES — Lymph nodes located in the area near the breastbone.

INTRADUCTAL — Residing within the duct of the breast. Intraductal disease may be benign or malignant.

INTRAVENOUS (I.V.) — Entering the body through a vein.

INVASIVE CANCER — Cancer that has spread outside of its site of origin and is growing into the surrounding tissues.

LATISSIMUS DORSI — Muscle tissue from the back used for breast reconstruction.

LESION — An area of tissue that is diseased.

LEUKOCYTE — A white blood cell or corpuscle.

LEUKOPENIA — A decrease in the number of white blood cells (where the count is less than 5,000); increases a person's susceptibility to infection.

LINEAR ACCELERATOR — A machine that produces high-energy X-ray beams to destroy cancer cells.

LIVER SCAN — A way of visualizing the liver by injecting into the bloodstream a trace dose of a radioactive substance which helps visualize the organ during X-ray.

LIVING WILL — Document signed by an individual stating her wishes in medical care issues if she is unable to properly communicate or make decisions.

LOBULAR — Pertaining to the part of the breast that is furthest from the nipple, the lobes.

LOCALIZED CANCER — A cancer still confined to its site of origin.

LOCAL RECURRENCE — Cancer that recurs in the area of the primary tumor, after a period of time when cancer was non-detectable, but has not spread to distant organs.

LUMPECTOMY — A surgical procedure in which only the cancerous tumor and an area of surrounding tissue are removed. Usually the surgeon will remove some of the underarm lymph nodes at the same time. This procedure is also referred to as a tylectomy.

LYMPH — A clear fluid circulating throughout the body in the lymphatic system that contains white blood cells and antibodies.

LYMPH NODES — Also called lymph glands. These are rounded body tissues in the lymphatic system that vary in size from a pinhead to an olive and may appear in groups or one at a time. The principal ones are in the neck, underarm and groin. These glands produce lymphocytes and monocytes (white blood cells which fight foreign substances) and serve as filters to prevent bacteria from entering the bloodstream. They will filter out cancer cells but will also serve as a site for metastatic disease. The major ones serving the breast are in the armpit. Some are located above and below the collarbone and some in between the ribs near the breast-bone. There are three levels of lymph nodes in the underarm area of the breast and another around the breastbone. The number of nodes varies from person to person. Lymph nodes are usually sampled during surgery to determine if the cancer has spread outside of the breast area.

LYMPHATIC VESSELS — Vessels that remove cellular waste from the body by filtering through lymph nodes and eventually emptying into the vascular (blood) system.

LYMPHEDEMA — A swelling in the arm (or extremities) caused by excess fluid that collects after the lymph nodes have been removed by surgery or affected by radiation treatments.

MAGNETIC RESONANCE IMAGING (MRI) — A magnetic scan; a form of X-ray using magnets instead of radiation. MRI gives a more clearly defined picture of fatty tissue than X-ray.

MALIGNANT TUMOR — A mass of cancer cells. These cells have uncontrolled growth and will invade surrounding tissues and spread to distant sites of the body, setting up new cancer sites; this process is called metastasis.

MARGINS — The area of tissue surrounding a tumor when the tumor is removed by surgery.

MASTECTOMY — Surgical removal of the entire breast, including nipple, areola, lymph nodes and some of the surrounding tissue.

- **MODIFIED RADICAL MASTECTOMY** — The most common type of mastectomy. Breast, breast skin, nipple, areola and underarm lymph nodes are removed. The chest muscles are saved.

- **PROPHYLACTIC MASTECTOMY** — A preventative procedure sometimes recommended for patients at a very high risk for developing cancer in one or both breasts.

- **RADICAL MASTECTOMY (HALSTED RADICAL)** — The surgical removal of the breast, breast skin, nipple, areola, chest muscles and underarm lymph nodes.

- **SEGMENTAL MASTECTOMY (PARTIAL MASTECTOMY/LUMPECTOMY)** — A surgical procedure in which only a portion of the breast is removed, including the cancer and the surrounding margin of healthy breast tissue.

- **SUBCUTANEOUS MASTECTOMY** — Performed before cancer is detected. A procedure that removes the breast tissue but leaves the outer skin, areola and nipple intact. (This is not suitable with a diagnosis of cancer.)

MENOPAUSE — The time in a woman's life when the menstrual cycle ends and the ovaries produce lower levels of hormones; usually occurs between the ages of 45 and 55.

METASTASIS — The spread of cancer from one part of the body to another through the lymphatic system or the bloodstream. The cells in the new cancer location are the same type as those in the original site.

MICROMETASTASIS — The undetectable spread of cancer outside of the breast that is not seen on routine screening tests. Metastasis is too limited to have created enough mass to be observed.

MITOTIC RATE — Rate of cell division and growth of a cancerous tumor.

MULTICENTRIC — Describes cancers or suspicious microcalcifications located over more than one quarter of the breast.

MULTIFOCAL — Describes cancers or suspicious microcalcifications located within one quarter of the breast.

MYELOSUPPRESSION — A decrease in the ability of the bone marrow cells to produce blood cells, including red blood cells, white blood cells and platelets. This condition increases susceptibility to infection, increases risk of bleeding and produces fatigue.

NADIR — The time after chemotherapy when blood cell counts reach their lowest levels. According to the type of blood cells affected by different drugs, an increase in infection, fatigue and bleeding may occur.

NECROSIS — Death of a tissue.

NEGATIVE NODES — Lymph nodes that do not have evidence of cancer after surgical removal and pathological evaluation.

NEO-ADJUVANT CHEMOTHERAPY — Chemotherapy given before surgery to treat breast cancer.

NEOPLASM — Any abnormal growth. Neoplasms may be benign or malignant, but the term usually is used to describe a cancer.

NEUTROPENIA – Low blood count values of neutrophil cells (type of white blood cells that fight infection); increases potential for infections.

NUCLEAR GRADE — An evaluation of the size and shape of the nucleus in tumor cells and the percentage of tumor cells that are in the process of dividing or growing.

ONCOGENE — Certain stretches of cellular DNA. Genes that, when inappropriately activated, contribute to the malignant transformation of a cell.

ONCOLOGIST — A physician who specializes in cancer treatment.

ONCOLOGY — The science dealing with the physical, chemical and biological properties and features of cancer, including causes, the disease process and therapies.

ONCOTYPE DX® — Test performed by evaluating 21 known genes in tumor cells of women with early stage breast cancer to evaluate the potential for breast cancer recurrence and need for chemotherapy.

OOPHORECTOMY — The surgical removal of the ovaries, sometimes performed as a part of therapy for breast cancer to reduce hormonal stimulation.

ORGASM — A state of physical and emotional excitement that occurs at the climax of sexual intercourse.

PATHOLOGIST — A physician with special training in diagnosing diseases from samples of tissue under a microscope.

PATHOLOGY — The study of disease through the microscopic examination of body tissues and organs. Any tumor suspected of being cancerous must be diagnosed by pathological examination.

PECTORALIS MUSCLES — Muscular tissues attached to the front of the chest wall and extending to the upper arms. These are under the breast and are divided into the pectoralis major and the pectoralis minor muscles.

PEDICLE FLAP — Tissues to reconstruct the breast that are taken from another area of the body, such as the stomach, buttocks or back, and remain attached to their original blood supply.

PER ORALLY (P.O.) — To take a medication by mouth.

PERMANENT SECTION — A technique in which a thin slice of biopsy tissue is mounted on a slide to be examined under a microscope by a pathologist in order to establish a diagnosis.

PLATELET — A cell formed by the bone marrow and circulating in the blood that is necessary for blood clotting. Platelet transfusions are used in cancer patients to prevent or control bleeding when the number of platelets has decreased.

PLOIDY — The number of chromosome sets in a cell.

PORT, LIFE PORT, PORT-A-CATH — A device surgically implanted under the skin, usually on the chest, that enters a large blood vessel and is used to deliver medication, chemotherapy, and blood products. Also used to obtain blood samples.

A port is usually inserted if a person has veins in the arm that are difficult to use for treatment or if certain types of chemotherapy drugs are to be given.

POSITIVE NODES — Lymph nodes removed during surgery that have cancer cells present after being studied by a pathologist.

PRECANCEROUS — Abnormal cellular changes that are potentially capable of becoming cancer. These early lesions are very amenable to treatment and cure. Also called pre-malignant.

PRETREATMENT MULTIDISCIPLINARY CONFERENCE — Meeting and discussion attended by different types of physicians involved in the treatment of breast cancer. Usually attended by a radiologist, surgeon, oncologist, radiation oncologist, reconstructive surgeon, genetic counselor, nurse navigator and other healthcare providers. Individual case is presented to the group after a positive biopsy and before any surgical intervention or treatment is started. Group discussion allows all physicians to offer their best clinical advice on the particular case under review before any final treatment decision is made.

PRIMARY TUMOR — First or original site of a cancer.

PROGESTERONE — Female hormone produced by the ovaries during a specific time in the menstrual cycle. Causes the uterus to prepare for pregnancy and the breasts to get ready to produce milk.

PROGESTERONE RECEPTOR ASSAY (PRA) — A test that is done on cancerous tissue to see if a breast cancer is progesterone hormone dependent and can be treated by hormonal therapy.

PROGESTERONE RECEPTORS (PR) — A receptor protein in breast cells to which progesterone will attach. Breast cancer cells that are PR+ depend on the hormone progesterone to grow and usually respond to hormonal therapy.

PROGNOSIS — A prediction of the course of the disease—the predicted future for the patient. For example, most breast cancer patients who receive treatment early have a good prognosis.

PROTOCOL — A schedule of selected drugs and treatment time intervals known to be effective against a certain cancer.

QUACKERY — Treatments, drugs or devices that claim to prevent, diagnose or cure diseases or health conditions, including cancer, that are known to be false or have no proven scientific evidence on which to base their claims.

RADIATION ONCOLOGIST — A physician specifically trained in the use of high energy X-rays to treat cancer.

RADIATION THERAPY — Treatment with high energy X-rays to destroy cancer cells.

RADIOLOGIST — A physician who specializes in diagnosing diseases by the use of X-rays.

RADIOTHERAPY — Treatment of cancer with high-energy radiation. Radiation therapy may be used to reduce the size of a cancer before surgery or to destroy any remaining cancer cells after surgery. Radiotherapy can be helpful in shrinking recurrent cancer to relieve symptoms such as pain and pressure.

RECONSTRUCTION — The rebuilding of the breast mound after surgical removal. Surgery performed by a reconstructive surgeon using implants or body tissues.

RECURRENCE — Reappearance of cancer after a period of remission.

REGIONAL INVOLVEMENT — The spread of cancer from its original site to nearby surrounding areas. Regional cancers are confined to one location of the body. Regional involvement in breast cancer could include the spread to the lymph nodes or to the chest wall.

RELAPSE — The reappearance of cancer after a disease-free period.

RELATIVE RISK REDUCTION — Figures derived by taking the absolute number of women benefiting from a therapy and translating it into a percentage of increase or decrease.

REMISSION — Complete or partial disappearance of the signs and symptoms of disease in response to treatment. The period during which a disease is under control. A remission, however, is not necessarily a cure.

S PHASE — A test that is performed to determine how many cells within the tumor are in a stage of division.

SARCOMA — A form of cancer that arises in the supportive tissues such as bone, cartilage, fat or muscle.

SECONDARY SITE — A second site in which cancer is found. Example: cancer in the lymph nodes near the breast is a secondary site.

SECONDARY TUMOR — A tumor that develops as a result of metastasis or spreads beyond the original cancer.

SENTINEL LYMPH NODE MAPPING — A procedure used to identify the first nodes draining a cancerous tumor by injecting a dye or radioactive contrast agent.

SENTINEL NODE(S) — First identified node or nodes that drain lymphatic fluid from a cancerous tumor.

SERMs (SELECTIVE ESTROGEN RECEPTOR MODULATORS) — Antihormonal drugs that can slow down or stop the growth of cancers that need estrogen to grow. Drugs in this group include tamoxifen, toremifene and raloxifene.

SEROMA — Collection of fluid (noncancerous) under the skin that feels soft and spongy.

SIDE EFFECTS — Usually describes situations that occur after treatments. For example, hair loss may be a side effect of chemotherapy; fatigue may be a side effect of radiation therapy.

SSRIs (SELECTIVE SEROTONIN REUPTAKE INHIBITORS) — A class of drugs that increase serotonin in the brain. Used in the treatment of depression.

STAGING — An evaluation of the extent of a disease, such as breast cancer. A classification based on stage at diagnosis which helps determine the appropriate treatment and prognosis. In breast cancer, the classification is determined by whether the lymph nodes are involved; whether the cancer has spread to other parts of the body (through the lymphatic system or bloodstream) and set up distant metastasis; and the size of the tumor. Five different stages (0 – 4) are used in breast cancer with levels in each stage. Stage IV is the most serious.

SUBCUTANEOUS (S.Q. OR S.C.) — To receive a medication by needle injection into the fatty tissues of the body.

SUPRACLAVICULAR NODES — The nodes located above the collarbone in the area of the neck.

SYSTEMIC — Pertaining to the whole body.

TAMOXIFEN — Anti-estrogen drug that may be given to women with estrogen receptive tumors to block estrogen from entering the breast tissues. May produce menopause-like symptoms, including hot flashes and vaginal dryness. Currently being used with high risk women in clinical trials to prevent breast cancer and with women who have had breast cancer to prevent recurrence.

TESTOSTERONE — Major male hormones found in lower amounts in females. Testosterone in females impacts and increases the sex drive and the ability to experience orgasm.

THROMBOCYTOPENIA — A decrease in the number of platelets in the blood, resulting in the potential for increased bleeding and decreased ability for clotting.

TRAM (TRANSVERSE RECTUS ABDOMINIS MUSCLE) — The tissue that is used to reconstruct a breast using the major stomach muscle attached to its original blood supply.

TREATMENT MODALITIES — Different types of treatment. For example: surgery, chemotherapy, radiation therapy and hormonal therapy.

TRIPLE NEGATIVE BREAST CANCER — Breast cancer that shows after testing that the tumor is receptor negative for estrogen (ER), progesterone (PR) and HER2 receptors (human epidermal growth factor receptor 2).

TUMOR — An abnormal tissue, swelling or mass; may be either benign or malignant.

TUMOR GROWTH RATE — Time required for a specific tumor to double in size. Same type of tumor may vary in growth rate from person to person.

U

ULTRASOUND EXAMINATION — The use of high frequency sound waves to locate a tumor inside the body. Helps determine if a breast lump is solid tissue or filled with fluids.

ULTRASOUND GUIDED BIOPSY — The use of ultrasound to guide a biopsy needle to obtain a sample of tissue for analysis by a pathologist.

W

WHITE BLOOD CELLS — Components of the blood, also known as leukocytes, that are able to kill bacteria and other invaders in the body. Low white blood cells—identified after a complete blood count is performed—causes one to be more susceptible to infections.

Index

lymph nodes 66–69, 72, 127, 218

M

margins 118, 219

mastectomy 72–76, 219–220

mood swings 151–152

N

neoadjuvant chemotherapy 66, 69, 132, 221

nipple reconstruction 94

node status 119

nuclear grade 119, 221

O

Oncotype DX® 132–133, 221

orgasm 168–170, 222

outpatient surgery 100–101

P

painful intercourse 170–172

pathologist 115, 222

pathology reports 115–129, 222

progesterone receptors (PR) 122–123, 223

prophylactic mastectomy 74, 220

R

radiation oncologist 134, 224

radiation therapy 134, 224

recommended reading 206–207

reconstruction/reconstructive surgery 79–97, 224

reconstruction complications 97

References

American Cancer Society Consumer's Guide to Cancer Drugs
Wilkes, G., R.N., M.S., A.O.C.N., and Ades, T., R.N., M.S., A.O.C.N.,
Sudbury, Massachusetts: Jones and Bartlett Publishers, 2000.

*The Breast: Comprehensive Management of Benign
and Malignant Disorders,* Third Edition
Bland, K., M.D., and Copeland, E., III, M.D., St. Louis: Elsevier Science, 2003.

Clinical Practice Guidelines in Oncology: Breast Cancer, Volume 1
National Comprehensive Cancer Network, 2009.
http://www.nccn.org/professionals/physician_gls/f_guidelines.asp.

Core Curriculum for Oncology Nursing
Itano, J., and Taoka, K., St. Louis: Saunders Company, 2005.

Diseases of the Breast, Third Edition
Harris, J., Lippman, M., Morrow, M., and Osborne, C.K.,
Philadelphia: Lippincott Williams & Wilkins, 2004.

Ferri's Clinical Advisor 2008: Instant Diagnosis and Treatment
Ferri, F., M.D., F.A.C.P., St. Louis: Mosby, 2008.

*Guidelines for Detection, Prevention and Risk Reduction:
Breast Cancer Risk Reduction,* Volume 1
National Comprehensive Cancer Network, 2009.
http://www.nccn.org/professionals/physician_gls/f_guidelines.asp.

*Guidelines for Detection, Prevention, and Risk Reduction: Genetic/Familial
High Risk Assessment Breast and Ovarian Cancer,* Volume 1
National Comprehensive Cancer Network, 2009.
http://www.nccn.org/professionals/physician_gls/f_guidelines.asp.

PDxMD: Hematology and Oncology
Ferrari, M., Britain: Elsevier Science, 2003.

Pocket Radiologist: Breast
Birdwell, R., M.D., Philadelphia: Saunders, 2003.

Psycho-oncology
Holland, J., M.D., New York: Oxford University Press, 1998.

Share the Gift of Understanding & Encouragement With Other Support Partners

♦ Would you like to help another support partner understand breast cancer and how to provide effective support for the one they love?

♦ Would you like to place this book in your local library as a gift from you?

♦ Would you like to give this book to the breast cancer treatment team to share with other support partners who are going through breast cancer treatment with someone they love?

You Can:

♦ Call Toll-Free: **1.800.849.9271**

♦ Order on the Web: **www.breasthealthcare.com**

Book(s) will be mailed to you or your selected recipient.

Price per book: $14.95 plus shipping

Price per book for 20 copies: $12.70 plus shipping

For larger quantity discounts with free customization, please call.

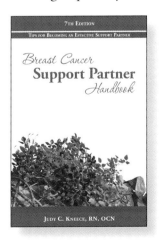

The role of a support partner is one of the most important components for the emotional recovery of a breast cancer patient.

Share the Gift of Hope

♦ Would you like to help a breast cancer patient regain her control by learning about her disease and what she can do to manage her emotions and enhance her recovery?

♦ Would you like to place this book in your local library as a gift from you?

♦ Would you like to give this book to the breast cancer treatment team to share with other patients going through treatment?

You Can:

♦ Call Toll-Free: **1.800.849.9271**

♦ Order on the Web: **www.breasthealthcare.com**

Book(s) will be mailed to you or your selected recipient.

Price per book: $24.95 plus shipping

Price per book for 20 copies: $20.95 plus shipping

For larger quantity discounts with free customization, please call.

The best weapon against breast cancer is an informed woman, working as a partner with her healthcare team.

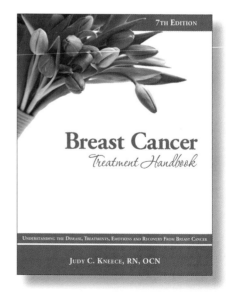

7TH EDITION

Breast Cancer
Treatment Handbook

UNDERSTANDING THE DISEASE, TREATMENTS, EMOTIONS AND RECOVERY FROM BREAST CANCER

JUDY C. KNEECE, RN, OCN